Every Voice Counts

Primary care organisations and public involvement

Will Anderson, Dominique Florin, Stephen Gillam and Lesley Mountford

The King's Fund is an independent charitable foundation working for better health, especially in London. We carry out research, policy analysis and development activities, working on our own, in partnerships, and through grants. We are a major resource to people working in health, offering leadership and education courses; seminars and workshops; publications; information and library services; a specialist bookshop; and conference and meeting facilities.

Published by
King's Fund
11–13 Cavendish Square
London W1G 0AN
www.kingsfund.org.uk

© King's Fund 2002

Charity registration number: 207401

First published 2002

ISBN 1 85717 460 7

A CIP catalogue record for this book is available from the British Library

Available from:
King's Fund Bookshop
11–13 Cavendish Square
London W1G 0AN
Tel: 020 7307 2591
Fax: 020 7307 2801
www.kingsfundbookshop.org.uk

Edited by Caroline Pook with Kita George
Cover design by Minuche Mazumdar Farrar
Typeset by Peter Powell Origination and Print Limited
Printed and bound in Great Britain

Contents

Acknowledgements

It is difficult to undertake research within busy primary care organisations without getting in the way, especially if the focus of the research is a hard-pushed agenda item such as public involvement. We are therefore very grateful to the many people who supported the study in the six London primary care organisations we worked with, who not only gave up their time for interviews but also welcomed us into the heart of their discussions and decision-making.

Thanks to the members, officers and many local stakeholders of Central Croydon Primary Care Group, City and Hackney Primary Care Trust, Dagenham Primary Care Group, Harrow East and Kingsbury Primary Care Group, Hayes and Harlington Directorate (Hillingdon Primary Care Trust) and North Lewisham Primary Care Group. We also acknowledge the important contributions made by North and South Croydon Primary Care Groups, Hillingdon Primary Care Trust as a whole and South Lewisham Primary Care Group.

Thanks to the GPs, practice nurses and many other health professionals who contributed to the study, and to the staff, members and volunteers of the community health councils, patient and public forums, voluntary organisations and community organisations in the six sites.

In particular, we would like to thank: Jean Atkinson, Nick Bailey, Derek Balaam, Elizabeth Bayliss, Geraldine Blake, Sandra Bodle, Mary Bond, Ping Bowman, Debbie Breen, Catherine Burns, Mary Cannon, Dr Velu Chandran, Mike Chapman, Mary Clarke, Lisa Clough, Kirsty Collander-Brown, Lucy Darlow, Geraint Davies, Anna Donovan, Malcolm Ellis, Samantha Flanders, Mary Flatley, Joanna Fox, Errol Franklin, Sue Gentry, Dr Ghosh, Bali Gill, Jill Godfrey, Amanda Gosling, Dr Clare Highton, Patricia Holmwood, Philip Hurst, Martin Hyams, Mohamed Ibrahim, Barbara Landey, Dr Jane Leaver, Brian Lymbery, Antonia Makinde, Joyce Mallagh, Anita Maynard, Fiona Millar, Jane Miller, Patricia Miller, Dr Akber Mohamedali, Helen Moroney, Dr Chaand Nagpaul, Anna O'Brien, Sharon Paradine, Alan Peel, Cathy Pelican, Rosemary Philbert, Margaret Philpot, Janett Plummer, Sarah Pond, Sidney Ramel, Deborah Richards, Janet Richardson, Phillippa Robinson, Maureen Sango-Jackson, Hilary Scarnell, Dr Gurdas Sethi, Paramjit Sethi, Laura Sharpe, Jess Steele, Doreen Stevens, Darshan Sundaram, Dr Gaby Tobias, Dr Alex Trumpetas, Peter Walsh, Sandy Walton, Sue Ward and Debbie Wickett.

For their encouragement and insight, thanks to the members of the steering group for the study: Maria Duggan, Brian Fisher and Ros Levenson. Thanks also to the support and enthusiasm of colleagues at the King's Fund, especially the members of the Primary Care Programme and the library team.

This was one of twelve studies into patient and public involvement funded by the *Health in Partnership* Programme of the Department of Health. We acknowledge the support of the Department, particularly the contributions of Dr Carolyn Davies, Christine Farrell and Dione Hills.

Will Anderson, Dominique Florin, Stephen Gillam and Lesley Mountford.

Summary of key findings

Drivers

Public involvement is principally value-driven.
People pursue it because they believe both in the
process – of listening, openness and dialogue – and in
its broad outcomes. It is rarely pursued either for its
own sake or simply as a means to an end.

See *Why bother?* page 11

Scope

Public involvement is about relationships. A focus on
methods in defining the scope of public involvement
can undervalue the many relationships that
institutions sustain with public voices. Activity
which is not part of the dialogue, but which enables
the dialogue (such as information/education and
community development) is sensibly included on
public involvement agendas.

See *What counts as public involvement?* page 15

Aims and outcomes

The development of corporate approaches to public
involvement is usually a negotiation. Different
stakeholders (inside and outside the organisation)
have different ideas about what public involvement
can achieve, and for whom. In this negotiation,
consensus about methods is often achieved without
clear agreement about what they are for.

See *What do you want to achieve?* page 19

This need not be an obstacle. In practice, the
outcomes of public involvement work are wide-
ranging, complex and often unexpected. An
approach which sustains a broad vision of the
potential of public involvement is more likely to
value this diversity of outcomes than an approach
which sticks to rigid goals. Discussion of aims should
not merely be a starting point, but part of on-going
reflection on practice.

Partnership

Partnership approaches to public involvement have
many potential benefits, particularly for primary care
organisations with a responsibility for their entire
local population. Expertise, knowledge and resources
can be shared, and duplication avoided. As public
perspectives do not respect institutional boundaries,

See *Turning to others* page 30

learning from public voices can be shared across health economies. But partnership is not cheap – working together, rather than simply talking together, takes time, effort and patience.

Requirements

A sustained public involvement programme is likely to require corporate commitment, leadership, significant resources and a clear strategy. But some progress in public involvement is possible with much less. Individual enthusiasm and basic executive support are the only absolute essentials. Corporate commitment may be necessary to long-term goals, but in practice this will only be built through corporate exposure to the value of public involvement.

See *Corporate essentials?* page 36

Voice

The choice of whom to involve will always be difficult. Reaching the many excluded voices in a health economy takes investment, sensitivity and patience. However, strong voices must also be valued – individuals who seek stronger voices though collective action or institutional roles should not lose credibility as a result. Whatever the form of engagement, there is always a tension between institutional and lay agendas. Both have to be valued for dialogue to succeed.

See *Who – and whose agenda?* page 43

Change

NHS organisations are not designed to learn from public voices. Public involvement work will achieve little if investment in methods of involvement is not matched by attention to internal mechanisms of learning and change.

See *Making a difference* page 55

Formal decision-making processes only take public views seriously if there are strong advocates for those views within them. However, organisations and their members and officers are open to influence in many other informal ways, which public voices should exploit. Whatever the approach, change is only likely if public involvement work connects in some way to existing organisational interests, where change is already on the agenda.

Chapter one

Introduction

This report is based on a study of six primary care organisations in London, conducted over 16 months from February 2000 to June 2001. When the study began, all six organisations were primary care groups (PCGs); when it finished, half of them had turned into primary care trusts (PCTs) and the rest were well on the way.

The study explored the development of public involvement work in these primary care organisations. 'Public involvement' is used as a short-hand throughout this book to encompass all forms of institutional and professional engagement with lay people – patients, carers, local people, local communities – other than the individual professional-patient relationship. We looked at everything from the role of the lay member on primary care group boards to community outreach.

This report attempts to capture the diversity of what we found. It also attempts to describe the practice of public involvement in a way that is useful to readers who are trying to get to grips with public involvement in primary care organisations.

This is not a comprehensive account of public involvement. Although our six case studies were very diverse, there were plenty of things that did not happen in any of them. There are no descriptions here of citizens' juries, rapid appraisal or electronic polling. There are a number of existing guides and tool-kits which do this job very well (see page 67). This publication is not a tool-kit, but an exploration of what shapes the development, implementation and outcomes of public involvement work. It draws attention to the importance of thinking about local circumstances, local people and local values as well as the detail of methods.

This report explores public involvement from the perspective of primary care organisations. Hopefully, many of the findings will be relevant to people elsewhere in the NHS and beyond. However, there are other very different stories to tell about public involvement in the NHS, from the perspectives of patients, carers, communities and the voluntary sector. As this publication does not tell these stories, we acknowledge their importance and the limitations of the stories told here.

As our title suggests, this publication is not value-free. We think that public involvement is a good thing. However, we hope that this report promotes a critical approach to public involvement, with an emphasis on delivering change. Public involvement is of little value if it goes nowhere – or if it is merely an exercise in public relations. But nor is it simply a means to an end.

Public involvement is a form of dialogue, of uncovering and valuing difference. This seems to us to be worthwhile, wherever it may lead.

Chapter two

Six case studies

The six primary care organisations in the study adopted strikingly different approaches to public involvement. The brief case descriptions over the next six pages focus on characteristic features of each, drawing attention to this diversity.

We have not attempted to give comprehensive accounts of what each organisation did. In these case descriptions, and in the further case details scattered through the rest of the book, we have highlighted the features of local practice which are most likely to be interesting and helpful to others.

It is worth bearing in mind the circumstances of these case studies. These were not well-established organisations with solid corporate identities. In February 2000, when we began, primary care groups had been in existence for less than a year. Although some drew on earlier experience as commissioning pilots, they were all struggling to pull together the basics of corporate infrastructure. For most primary care professionals, steeped in the history of independent practice, corporate life was itself a radical change.

Thrust into the driving seat of the new NHS, primary care professionals also had to struggle with a huge agenda of change. There was work to do on every front. Not surprisingly, public involvement proved to be one of many priorities (see below).

As researchers, we sought to be both flexible and helpful. We began with interviews with key stakeholders in each primary care organisation, but most of the research involved observation and participation in planning meetings, board meetings and specific public involvement initiatives.

For a fuller account of the methods used, see the appendix on page 78.

One of many priorities: public involvement in primary care groups

Anderson W and Florin D. London: King's Fund, 2000.

This report describes the results of a survey of lay members and chief officers of primary care groups, undertaken in October 1999, which informed the selection of these case studies.

Although 76 per cent of chief executives said that developing public involvement was a 'high priority', there were many other high priorities. Out of 13 key concerns, developing public involvement came ninth, with only 16 per cent identifying this as higher then their average 'high priority'. Their highest priorities were establishing infrastructure, developing primary care and financial management.

Central Croydon

Central Croydon PCG did not lack ambition. With the support of the local community health council and Croydon Voluntary Action (CVA), they set out to create a distinct approach to public involvement that would join up their own corporate interests with those of patients in local practices and the community/voluntary sector.

The result was a substantial standing mechanism, supported by CVA, which brought all these stakeholders together in a regular community forum. The forum was chaired by a CVA worker with the lay member and officers from the PCG presenting papers from the board for discussion. It was also attended by individual link patients from some of the local practices and by members of local voluntary organisations – and members of the public.

The link people were a crucial part of the scheme. Most had their own notice boards within their practices where they displayed information from the PCG. And, as far as they could, they tried to identify practice-based concerns to take to the community forum and to the PCG officers.

Inevitably, this grand scheme had its problems. Some of the link people felt isolated and unsupported by practice staff. The CVA worker did not have adequate time to address the needs of the link people while also servicing the community forum. There was not enough time in the forums themselves to address all the issues which people wanted to talk about. The officer who presented PCG papers to forum was often unable to answer all the detailed questions that were raised.

Like most grand schemes, it took on a life of its own. The people who got involved in it invested different interests in it and got different things out of it. It worked, to an extent, for everyone – but in different ways. The lay member wanted the forums to inform her own contributions to the board as a lay representative. The officer wanted the forum and link people to be the key means of communication with local practices. The CVA worker wanted the whole scheme to operate as community development, enabling participants to gain confidence and act collectively.

The individual link people gained a lot from the forums through hearing about local health services and participating in debate with officers, members and their own peers. However, many also wanted to influence PCG policy, and this seemed the hardest goal to achieve. There were formal links between the forum and the board, but the board only met four times a year and most of the decision-making took place elsewhere. It was hard for them to know how much difference they were really making.

Central Croydon's ambition to create a substantial standing process for public involvement was realised. Having created it, they faced the considerable on-going challenge of keeping all its moving parts well-oiled and properly balanced. It would not be easy to keep everyone on board if it delivered for some but not for others.

City & Hackney

In March 2000, Hackney PCG held its last board meeting. Within a week it would be a gleaming new primary care trust. At this meeting, the chief officer of the community health council congratulated the members of the board on the changes they had brought to the local health economy.

There had been no transformation in service provision and the impact of the organisation on the health of the population had probably been marginal. Yet the PCG had replaced defensiveness and secrecy with openness and trust. They had been honest about what they could and could not do. And this honesty was the foundation of a new local spirit of partnership – other local stakeholders felt that their voices would be taken seriously, even if there was little scope for the PCG to address everything which these local voices wanted to raise.

Hackney's public involvement work was driven by an understanding that the PCG could not promote the health of a highly deprived local population by putting its head down and getting on with the job. It had to open up to all the other organisations and people in the community who also had a part to play in promoting health – potentially every group, every patient, every citizen, every worker. Following the lead of a committed chief officer, considerable energy was devoted to going to meet local community groups on their own turf, building relationships with key individuals and enabling communication. At the same time, new formal structures were developed for voluntary sector involvement in strategic planning and commissioning. As well as going out to listen to the community, the PCG ensured that the confident voices in the community were heard when its own agenda was on the table.

The PCG struggled to exploit these new relationships. There was too much to do and too few resources. The PCG's community participation steering group, chaired by the lay member, brought people together from across the health economy to build a common vision of public involvement, but there was inadequate officer support to turn its aspirations into action. An imaginative PCT consultation involving extensive outreach with community groups produced recommendations for change which ended up on no officer's 'to do' list. The lay member kept the profile of community participation high on the board's agenda, but did not have the resources to follow through across the detail of the PCG's daily business.

The PCG had built a culture of partnership and trust, a good foundation for its new life as an autonomous trust. It now faced the challenge of fulfilling some of the expectations created in this new environment.

Dagenham

When the lay member attended her first meeting of Dagenham PCG, she was not introduced, her skills went unrecognised and her voice was ignored. It seemed unlikely that the small business ethic which dominated the PCG would make any room for her community-focussed values.

But there were other people who shared her values, who were committed to listening to and working with local people. A public involvement subgroup was soon established, which brought together a varied group of people with a common interest in building the bridges between professionals, patients, carers, and the communities where they worked. The group met in the surgery of the one local GP who really saw the point of public involvement. A key member of the subgroup was the chair of the patient participation group (PPG) based there.

The PCG group did not proceed in an orderly fashion. It was not merely a planning group, but an opportunity for its members to debate, reflect on their practice and let off steam. Although it lacked clear leadership, the group was sustained by a shared commitment to improving the quality of local primary care through closer partnership with patients and carers.

As the PPG was the only clear example of local success in public involvement in primary care, it became the focus of a development programme for other practices in the area. The chair of the PPG and the lay member encouraged other local GPs to develop similar groups. Unfortunately, this proved too ambitious: the subgroup had spent too much time sharing ideals and too little time thinking through what was actually necessary to achieve their ideals. Subsequently, they took several steps back and invested instead in a training programme for primary care professionals in the basics of patient partnership.

The lay member's community values embraced a commitment to listening to everyone's voice, not just the strongest voices. This inspired the subgroup to plan a significant piece of qualitative research, designed to hear the voices of people who were highly dependent on services, as patients or carers – people who are usually too vulnerable to question the practice of their own providers. The research was conducted with the support of local voluntary organisations: confident voices enabling the PCG to get access to distant voices. The report from the study was powerful reading and the officer concerned felt confident that it addressed a number of the organisation's immediate interests. But she was left the difficult task of ensuring that the connections between these local voices and the institutional agenda were made.

When the lay member left the PCG, it had changed. Attitudes on the board had begun to shift, albeit slowly. And a precedent had been set for the PCT that lay and community voices did have a meaningful and valuable role in the corporate process.

Harrow East & Kingsbury

No-one in Harrow East & Kingsbury PCG knew much about public involvement. Nor did anyone in the local GP practices. The lay member was charged by the board with leading the PCG's public involvement work, but confessed that he had little idea of what this required. Other board members were happy to sign up to a hastily prepared public involvement strategy, but then paid it no more attention – and nor did anyone else.

Yet before they knew it, the PCG had a programme of public involvement underway. A small subgroup, convened by the lay member, rapidly realised that the PCG would have to look elsewhere for help. It therefore sought to tap into whatever local mechanisms were already established. The local authority had a citizens' panel, which seemed like a good opportunity. And the health authority had plans to run focus groups with local diabetics. So the subgroup agreed to use the citizens' panel for a survey of its own and to support the local implementation of the focus groups.

Although this approach appeared quite ad hoc, reaching out to whatever else was going on, there was consistency in the group's discussions about what they wanted to achieve. They were principally concerned with the quality of service delivery and the appropriateness of service design. However, they were also interested in the quality of their users' self-care and the appropriateness of their service use – i.e. with demand as well as of supply. Happily, both of the key methods they adopted could be used to further these interests.

The survey of the citizens' panel proved to be a more complicated task than the opportunity first suggested. Having chosen the method, the group had to work out what they wanted to do with it and what questions they wanted to ask. A questionnaire had to be designed and piloted; results had to be input, analysed and written up. Nonetheless, when the whole project was completed, it gave the PCG board a picture of local knowledge and priorities, which proved to be extremely timely for its own consideration of primary care development priorities.

The diabetic focus groups became seminars, run in a variety of local languages. Although these were more about giving information than listening, their popularity led to the creation of regular facilitated support groups for different local ethnic minority populations. Although there was no formal process of feeding back information to the PCG from these groups, the nurse in charge played a critical role in picking up on local concerns and taking them directly to the professionals in the PCG or its constituent practices, where action could be taken.

So, despite the lack of public involvement expertise within the PCG, and the failure to think through what was required to bring about change, they got results.

Hayes & Harlington

There was no doubt in Hayes & Harlington PCG that lay members were central to the task of public involvement. In fact, they decided to have two.

The two lay members were kept busy. They contributed to many of the subgroups as well as to the business of the board itself. They participated in a regular public forum, run by the community health council, which discussed PCG business with local patients. They visited a range of local community groups and associations to inform people about primary care services and to listen to their concerns.

Crucially, the lay members were heavily involved both as insiders, engaging with the detail of the organisation's business, and as outsiders, listening to the voices of patients and local people. It was therefore largely up to them to make the connections between the two.

On the face of it, this was difficult and the formal process did not look too good. The lay members took notes from the meetings, wrote them up and presented them to the board for discussion. But these notes could never capture the variety and passion of the original voices, and the board was never terribly interested, or simply too busy with more pressing papers.

However, the connections did get made. The board was never a great place for influence anyway – most of the decisions had already been made. The participation of the lay members in the subgroups gave them much more scope to influence the development of policy, drawing on their experience with local people. It was here that change was most likely.

The PCG did not, however, rely entirely on the lay members as conduits of patient and public voices. A community health council officer also played an important role in challenging the assumptions and decision-making of the board. Because she was much more of an outsider, she could ruffle more feathers than the lay members.

The public forum was most powerful when it did not rely on intermediaries. When the chair or chief officer of the PCG attended and engaged directly with the members of the forum, there was enormous scope for learning on both sides. There is nothing that beats considered, face-to-face dialogue as a process of learning and change for all concerned.

When the PCG became a PCT, it held on to its lay members, keeping them on the executive committee, where they were joined by the same community health council officer and a non-executive director seconded from the PCT board. Therefore there were four lay voices on a board that was not required to have any. Clearly, the value of corporate lay voices in aiding decision-making had been accepted.

North Lewisham

North Lewisham PCG had a wealth of local resources to draw on in developing its public involvement work: a community development project with a focus on primary care; officers and members with commitment and expertise; an active and supportive community health council; a diverse and well-organised voluntary sector; regeneration initiatives with strong community participation elements to them; a health authority with an established programme of involvement work; local investment through a Health Action Zone (HAZ) in health-focussed community development.

The difficulty for the PCG was therefore to carve an appropriate role for its public involvement work within this complex context. It sought to do this by investing in the process of partnership. The principal responsibility of the officer who supported the public involvement work was the development of local partnerships. In this way, partnership with patients and communities was supported through a broader process of partnership, which embraced statutory and voluntary sector interests. This was also reflected in the diverse membership of the PCG's public involvement subgroup, chaired by the lay member.

The PCG supported the community development project in promoting involvement at practice level, and worked with the voluntary sector and community health council to establish corporate means of listening to local people about their needs. It also sought to ensure that these and all other stakeholders could contribute to its own strategic development. The community development sponsored through the HAZ strengthened relationships between the voluntary/community sector and the PCG as well as relationships within the sector itself.

However, this beautifully integrated vision was still messy in practice. Although the PCG had some officer support for the work, it was very limited. So it proved difficult to maximise the potential of all these possibilities. There seemed to be lots going on, but no clear process of making the most of it all. This was expressed by some as a frustration with the inability of the PCG to be clear about how it actually used the knowledge it gained from the community. There was a lot of community intelligence around and still more was being generated. Yet the ways in which this intelligence was used and valued by the PCG was far from transparent.

The PCG was also overtaken by events. Considerable investment was made in the PCT consultation process and in a rapid consultation prior to the development of a local health centre. The more there was to do, the harder it was to keep everything joined up. The case for a dedicated worker, who could join up the public involvement work and connect it to the rest of the interests of the organisation, became overwhelming, and a new public co-ordinator was soon appointed.

Chapter three

Why bother?

KEY POINTS

Policy is rarely a direct driver of public involvement work unless it includes 'must dos'.

Public involvement work is value driven. Most people pursue it because they are committed to the process and its broad goals.

People are rarely persuaded solely by the 'business case' for public involvement, but rather by experience of public involvement in action.

The wide variety of values which sustain public involvement work include values of democracy, partnership, community and consumerism.

Commitment to broad goals does not resolve the tricky question of what to do in practice.

Why bother to pursue public involvement?

Well, for a start, it's policy. For the last ten years or more public involvement has been increasingly written into government health policy. It is no longer an option but a duty of the NHS to involve the public in the planning and development of services.

Of course, being part of policy is not a sufficient reason for pursuing public involvement. Doing it because it has to be done is exactly the sort of practice which infuriates people who are invited to participate. Ticking the public involvement box and doing no more is a waste of everyone's time.

But how much of a driver has policy been to local public involvement work? In our case studies, there was little evidence of direct effects. In only one of the primary care organisations had the arrival of new government guidance on public involvement inspired a significant response (see box right). In the others, such guidance had idiosyncratic, marginal effects – until the NHS Plan forced everyone to consider the future of their practice.

In City & Hackney, the 1999 guidance *Patient and Public Involvement in the new NHS* was briefly used by the community participation steering group because it offered a 'framework for assessing progress on patient and public involvement'. This seemed to provide a useful tool for describing local work but, even at this level, the imposition of a grid from elsewhere proved clumsy and insensitive to local values so it was eventually abandoned. The rest of the document was ignored – the group had enough to think about without having to worry about the NHSE's interpretations of what their agenda ought to be.

Elsewhere, the same document had a more significant impact: the Harrow East public involvement subgroup was set up at the end of 1999 explicitly in response to this guidance. As there was little existing activity or expertise within the organisation, there was much greater opportunity for central policy to have an impact. Ironically, however, the document did not give the group what it required – clear guidance about what to do. So the content of the document was soon forgotten as the group set about identifying existing local initiatives to tap in to.

Prior to the NHS Plan, there was only one piece of policy which had an important impact: the inclusion of lay members on primary care group boards. This was a 'must do', so everyone did it. Once appointed, the lay members found that the creation of their role was not followed by very clear guidance about what it actually involved, so they all had to work this out for themselves.

Lay members were important in all sorts of ways, explored throughout this publication. Simply by being there, by being a lay voice within professional debate, they forced their peers to consider the value of user and public voices in the board room as well as the consulting room. In their many contributions to the business of PCGs, lay members offered an answer to the question 'why bother?', though inevitably some provided a better answer than others.

What motivated local champions of public involvement was not policy, but what they believed in. Public involvement was, above all, driven by values. These values encompassed both the process of involvement – dialogue, partnership, communication – and its broad goals. Public involvement was rarely seen either as something worth doing just for its own sake or simply as a means to an end.

There were times when people felt that they had to emphasise the 'business case' for public involvement, i.e. purely instrumental arguments. This, typically, was when they had to persuade people who did not share their basic values. However, this business case is rarely very persuasive to people who are wary in the first place. Winning people over takes time and experience – people usually need to see values in action before they come round to them. In all our case studies, there was some culture change in this direction as primary care professionals learnt to work with lay members and engage in broader partnership with local communities.

The values which sustain public involvement work are remarkably diverse. They are described here as four broad types: the values of democracy, partnership, community and consumerism.

For some people, public involvement stands as a value in itself, something all statutory bodies should

In City & Hackney, the lay member wanted to sustain a broad vision of working in partnership across the local community in which everyone's voice was valued. However, she accepted that this vision was too long on process and too short on outcomes for the hard-nosed and hard-pressed GPs in the PCG. So she tried to make a more pragmatic case for public involvement in simple ways, for example by getting the health gains of self-care written into the Health Improvement Programme.

In Dagenham, a diverse range of values sustained the discussions in the public involvement subgroup, but the fragile state of local primary care also concentrated their minds on a very specific outcome: better services. They wanted to be clear, to each other and to the professionals around them, that greater patient partnership within practices would not create trouble but bring benefits for everyone involved.

I think there is a tone of honesty, starting at board level and chair level and at my level, that means you don't have to try and cover things up and make it seem all right at the time. You can actually acknowledge all of it and that takes a lot of heat out of the system. So for me that's critical.

Chief officer

seek to achieve. However, this is always linked to other values of accountability, transparency, openness and trust. These are democratic values which focus on the relationships between patients and providers, citizens and institutions.

Unfortunately, democratic values are difficult to nurture in the inward looking, risk-averse bureaucracy of the NHS. The NHS was not designed to be democratic, and the small business culture of primary care is not a good starting point for change. Holding board meetings in public is one thing; promoting a culture of openness is quite another. Although many of the individuals involved in our case studies believed in these values, only two of the primary care organisations made explicit corporate commitments to them.

If relationships are at the heart of democratic values, they also inspire a wider set of values – of partnership and shared responsibility for common goals. People who believe in the value of partnership are likely to see public involvement as an opportunity to bring in patients, carers and local people into the shared task of promoting health. Again, these are not familiar values to primary care. Working in partnership was widely accepted as a value by individuals in our case studies but treated with suspicion by many professional board members who perceived the costs of partnership but not the benefits.

The value of partnership takes us to the wider community in which primary care organisations operate. Is this community a source of problems which professionals have to address or a source of intelligence and skills in dealing with local health problems? This defines a set of communitarian values which inspired public involvement work. Many of the most committed individuals in our case studies were the people who believed in their communities, who wanted to work with communities because they were a source of strength, and a resource in the task of health improvement. This was a real challenge to many professionals whose view of the community was dominated by the endless stream of needy patients arriving in their consulting rooms.

Finally, there are consumer values, focussed on the priority of delivering services which are sensitive to

We're very exposed to public criticism and comment because if things go wrong lives can be threatened; so there is inevitably the sort of culture in the health service which doesn't want people to take risks because sometimes inevitably taking risks or even going out on a limb a bit can lead to things going wrong. And if things go wrong there's all hell to pay. And I feel that sometimes the approach therefore is not 'What can we do to make this better?' but 'How can we avoid things going wrong while we're making it better?'

Lay member

Well obviously I'm a local girl so I've always had this philosophy that you should give back to your community something that you take out. One of the things I as an individual truly believe in is that services are better focused on the local community. So that was the reason why I applied.

Lay member

In Dagenham, the contrast between professional and community values was marked. The lay member brought to the board a commitment to listening to and working with local people which was barely acknowledged by most of her professional peers. The dominant values of the board reflected the small business ethos of the GPs, which did not sit easily with a vision of working in partnership with local people to meet local needs. Nonetheless, the strength of the lay member's commitment ensured that the PCG invested in a process of listening to, and learning from, local primary care users, whose views about service provision had traditionally been ignored.

individual needs and wants. Although these values have been very prominent in national policy, they were dominant in only one of our case studies. Across all the case studies, there was an understanding that public involvement ought to be part of the process of service development. But public involvement was rarely seen simply as a form of market research.

What all these values mean in practice is another matter. Values shape broad goals but not specific operational aims and objectives. They provide motivation and general direction, but the task of working out the best way forward, given the complicated map of local circumstances, remains.

Chapter four

What counts as public involvement?

KEY POINTS

Definitions of public involvement are never final – they are always being renegotiated as people come and go within local discussions.

If public involvement is defined too narrowly, as a collection of methods rather than a range of relationships, existing practice can be undervalued.

Every public voice has a value, including those of voluntary organisations, institutional representatives and staff (who are patients and carers too).

Information and education are a necessary if not sufficient part of public involvement work and are sensibly included on public involvement agendas.

Public involvement is not community development, but strong community voices are invaluable to public involvement work.

Public involvement is a mixed bag. There are all sorts of different things which are described as public involvement. There are also different opinions about what should be in the bag and what should be left out.

Perhaps this does not matter very much, as long as the people who develop public involvement work reach their own consensus about what they are doing. In practice, what gets on local public involvement agendas is always a negotiation between the individuals involved, and so changes as people come and go.

Nonetheless, there is a danger that public involvement is defined, explicitly or implicitly, too narrowly. In particular, the emphasis in much discussion of public involvement on specific methods leads to forgetfulness that public involvement is about relationships, and that relationships can be sustained in ways other than through 'tool-kit' methods. Does lifting the phone on a Friday afternoon and ringing the director of the local Age Concern to discuss a policy paper count as public involvement? If not, why not?

If public involvement is defined narrowly, existing practice may be under-valued or simply ignored.

In Harrow East & Kingsbury, the chair, chief officer and lay member all felt overwhelmed by the public involvement agenda and did not know where to take their first bite out of the 'elephant sandwich'. Yet they were already heavily involved in a local partnership through which officers regularly came into contact with representatives of voluntary organisations to discuss strategic health issues. This was not included on their public involvement group's agenda, which struggled to develop new interventions which would demonstrate their commitment to public involvement.

In Hayes & Harlington, public involvement was strongly identified with the lay members and the work they supported. Because the lay members were people with a voice inside the organisation, other members and officers had to engage with the idea of public involvement as a relationship – as people they had to talk to on a regular basis – as well as a lot of meetings or groups which they could happily ignore. However, this did not change the corporate view that public involvement was principally something which the lay members and community health council did, and not something which other officers and members engaged in on a day-to-day basis.

Primary care organisations that treat public involvement as a 'new' agenda item can all too easily begin the task by ignoring everything they are already doing.

In our case studies, public involvement did take quite different directions in different places. This was largely because of different choices about what to prioritise within public involvement. In particular, two of the primary care organisations focussed almost entirely on the experience of users; whereas two of the others were mainly concerned with the interests of local communities. However, there were also differences across the case studies in what got on the public involvement agenda at all. The following were included on some agendas but were questioned (or disregarded) on others:

- voluntary sector partnership
- institutional lay representation
- staff involvement
- information and education
- community development.

In our case studies, the voluntary sector was never explicitly excluded from public involvement agendas, but partnership arrangements with the voluntary sector were not always perceived to be part of the public involvement brief. This typically reflects a perception that the voices of 'ordinary people' cannot be represented by voluntary organisations, or indeed by institutional lay members.

Such distinctions are unhelpful (see page 50), not least because they disempower individuals who seek to gain confidence through joining collective voices. Similarly, the institutional lay member who puts great effort into understanding the internal agenda of an organisation is ill-served if this is used to question the 'authenticity' of their lay perspective.

Staff involvement is the final frontier of this problem. Surely people who work for an organisation cannot also speak for the organisation's users? But what if they are themselves a patient, mother, carer or local resident – is this all deemed irrelevant because of their professional interests? Staff involvement is normally treated as a separate policy issue from public involvement, because of its focus on

In City & Hackney an explicit attempt was made to acknowledge the potential role of staff, particularly frontline staff, in the public involvement process. This was three-fold: first, many staff were themselves local residents who had personal experience of how local conditions impacted on health; second, all staff were potentially patients or carers with their own understanding of the problems of using health services; and third, in their professional roles, frontline staff gained enormous intelligence about the needs of local people. By thinking of public involvement as a broad process of engaging with local communities and seeking intelligence about local needs, the potential for staff to play a key role in the process was recognised.

professional interests. However, there is plenty of scope to overcome such divides and value the contribution of staff, both as public voices in their own right and as conduits to public voices in their professional roles.

Information and education are often considered not to count as 'involvement' because the relationship is completely one-sided – the organisation learns nothing. They are right at the bottom of Arnstein's ladder of participation (see box over). Nonetheless, it makes practical sense for information to be on public involvement agendas. All public involvement work includes some aspect of information-giving, and information and education are part of the process of enabling individuals and organisations to participate in health service decision-making. A public involvement group which only discussed information-giving might not be getting off the starting line, but it is also a mistake to undervalue the information and education outcomes for local people which public involvement work delivers.

Community development is as mixed a bag as public involvement. Although a distinction is usually drawn between community development and public involvement, there are obvious overlaps between the two. Public involvement work needs individuals and communities who can express their own interests and needs; community development increases the capacity of the community to do this. However, the tricky issue is whether this is what community development is for. A 'pure' form of community development would disregard organisational interests and focus on enabling the community to identify and address its own needs. But in practice, there are always connections between the two.

In the long term we have got to have a way of thinking about community participation that is much more sophisticated and multilevel and this understanding has got to be in the heads of practitioners and community staff, so that they understand that involving people is something that can be done in all sorts of different ways and it's a daily issue.

Community participation is about ownership of our public services, and the ownership includes the people who clean the offices as well as the people who run the hospital. Many of the people who work in our local public services live here, locally, and that difference between working in service and being a recipient of it is something artificial, certainly in an area like this.

Lay member

North Lewisham made the biggest commitment to community development, including a borough-wide co-ordinator (funded by HAZ) who worked with local community groups and organisations. However, it was not always clear if this officer's brief should be focussed entirely on enabling community organisations to be more effective in their own networks, or whether she should also be facilitating stronger relationships with the PCG, i.e. enabling the PCG's user and public involvement work. Community development was seen as a distinct process which could be undermined by poorly planned public involvement work if community organisations' expectations of meaningful relationships with statutory institutions were not met.

In City & Hackney, there was no such anxiety about the boundary between empowering and involving local communities. The focus of the community participation subgroup was as much on the resourcing and development of local communities as it was on involvement. This contributed to the group's difficulty in making progress: community empowerment is always long term.

A ladder of citizen participation

Arnstein S. *Journal of the American Planning Association* 1969;
vol. 35 no. 4: 216–224.

Arnstein's famous ladder of participation describes the power relationships between institutions and citizens.

The citizens start out powerless at the bottom of the ladder which is propped up against the institution where power resides. It is up to the institution to decide how far up the ladder the citizens can climb.

Arnstein defined eight levels of participation, but these are usually simplified to the following:

- At the bottom of the ladder, citizens have no say in what goes on, but are kept informed about decision-making. Information goes one way.

- On the next rung up, citizens are invited to respond to proposals, but the institution retains the decision-making role. This is consultation.

- A further step up, and the decision-making power is shared between the institution and citizens. This is partnership.

- Finally, on the top rung, the citizens take over the power of decision-making – citizen control.

The ladder is a useful tool for getting people to be upfront about their expectations. It is all too easy for statutory organisations to talk about partnership when they have no real intention of sharing decision-making power. This is not wrong – 'partnership' is a vague word which is used in many ways. But if no-one stops to explore what different people mean by it, someone is likely to end up disappointed. It is far better to do a good consultation than to offer partnership and then fail to deliver.

In our case studies, questions about the power relationships created through public involvement were rarely raised. This was partly because the immaturity of the work meant that much of it was necessarily focussed on information and consultation. However, it was also because people usually discussed their work in terms of the kinds of activity they wanted to engage in or what they wanted to achieve. They rarely made time for more analytical discussions about the nature of the power relations involved.

This ladder should be used with care. In practice, public involvement initiatives may continually shift between rungs, often in subtle and unexpected ways. Furthermore, the ladder only describes one aspect of relationships. Trust is critical to relationships, yet may be completely missing at any level on Arnstein's ladder. Even if the formal mechanisms are in place for sharing decision-making, genuine partnership is unlikely to exist without trust.

Chapter five

What do you want to achieve?

KEY POINTS

Corporate approaches to public involvement rarely have clear starting points. They emerge out of existing practice and commitments.

The planning of public involvement work is usually a negotiation between stakeholders with different priorities and interests. Agreement on methods may not indicate agreement on aims.

Aims are not merely a starting point: discussion of aims can happen at any time in the development and implementation of public involvement work.

The outcomes from public involvement work are often unexpected. Openness to the value of all outcomes contributes to the on-going renegotiation of aims.

Changes to professional and institutional practice can be hard to identify, either as goals and as outcomes, but commitment to seeing through the impact of public involvement to this level is crucial.

There are lots of things people hope to achieve through public involvement, such as better services, greater accountability, stronger communities and even a healthier population. The potential is perceived to be enormous.

Yet for all its potential, public involvement work often suffers from a lack of clarity about its aims. Aims may be defined too broadly, left unconnected to specific objectives, be disputed, or simply not be discussed. It is easy for public involvement methods to gain their own momentum and be pursued with no agreement about what they are trying to achieve. This chapter describes some of these problems, exploring:

- the complexity of the context in which public involvement is planned
- the negotiation which takes place in planning public involvement
- the differences between aims and outcomes in practice
- the importance of setting goals
- the range of potential goals for public involvement.

It's about being clear about what you are doing and being honest about that, not pretending that you are doing otherwise. So if you are disseminating information, be clear that that is what you are doing: you're not getting people's views, you're just giving them information. And when you're consulting with people you're being clear with them how far they can really influence policy.

Officer

A messy business

It is tempting, under this chapter heading, to prescribe the rational ideal: to insist that aims and objectives must be defined first; an approach refined; then implementation seen through, carefully monitored and evaluated; before the whole process starts again. But in reality, this almost never happens.

The world is simply too messy, and public involvement too messy a business, for a tidy progression from aims through methods to outcomes. An officer of a primary care organisation with an interest in pursuing public involvement is unlikely to be the only one locally with this interest. There will be other people with different values and ideas about what should be done and what it might be for. There will be various things going on already (initiatives, partnerships, networks) which, over time, may have fulfilled different interests and achieved a variety of outcomes. There are likely to be many potential stakeholders with different degrees of power, influence and commitment.

Given such diversity of existing interests and activity, there may be no clear starting point when everyone can sit down and decide their aims. This does not mean that aims are ignored. Rather, they become part of the on-going conversation – a point of reflection on practice, rather than the defining framework for practice.

In our case studies, none of the primary care organisations started life with a blank sheet for public involvement. Each sought to build on existing practice and experience in the local health economy. From the beginning, discussions were focussed as much on existing methods as on potential goals. Consequently, articulation of goals was as much driven by appreciation of existing practice as it was the driver for new initiatives.

Planning public involvement is an on-going negotiation

People who stick to the rational planning ideal are easily frustrated by public involvement work. The apparent failure of many discussions about public involvement to move clearly from aims to objectives

In Hayes & Harlington, there was already a history of public involvement work led by the community health council when the lay members joined the organisation. The CHC public panel had been set up with a broad remit to improve the accountability of the new primary care organisations. In practice, this meant that the panel participants spent a lot of time discussing board papers – focussing on corporate decision-making. As members of the board, the lay members had a similar interest. Consequently, the general consensus that public involvement was principally about influencing board decisions was a product both of local history and the peculiarity of the lay role (and the priority given to it here). However, the lay members were also keen to involve a wider range of people in the process and so began a series of community meetings: a clearer case of aims defining methods, rather than the other way round.

I don't know that anybody is completely sure what it is they are expecting to achieve because you're not going to suddenly get the community setting up primary care centres or something. We've got the voluntary sector and the residents associations in – really bringing them into the fold and running sessions for them. Well, it's better than a kick in the teeth, isn't it?

Public involvement worker

Designed to involve: public involvement in the new primary care structures

Scottish Office, Scottish Association of Health Councils, Scottish Consumer Council. Glasgow: Scottish Consumer Council, 1999.

This guide to developing public involvement in primary care trusts, sponsored by the Scottish Office, balances an understanding of the complexity of the task with a version of the traditional planning process. It acknowledges that:

'Planning for public involvement should be a dynamic process involving many partners. The development of participative work can be an educational process for organisations, patients, public representatives and communities. It can create new links, develop larger projects and collaborations from the successes of smaller ones, and from these build confidence in the ability of collaborative work to provide useful new policy directions and models.'

Their recommended planning cycle has five key elements:

- development of a vision, articulated in policy
- collaborative development of strategy
- audit of current practice
- development and support of a range of activities
- monitoring, evaluation and feedback.

This is a useful model for thinking through the components of strategic public involvement work. However, in our case studies, these tasks did not usually happen in regular 'phases', but were concurrent. Their relationships were also complex – for example, corporate vision was often weak at the outset but developed through experience of practice. Formal written strategies also served different purposes to the unwritten practical strategies in the heads of members and officers (see page 41).

to implementation suggests too muddled an approach with little hope of impact.

These may be reasonable concerns (see below), but we should not assume that there is only one effective approach to planning. Open-ended, exploratory approaches to public involvement in which there is an on-going dialogue about aims and outcomes, not least during the process of implementation, can also be effective – though what counts as success will itself be constantly reconsidered.

If this sounds woolly, consider the practice rather than the planning of public involvement. Public involvement is about the meeting of different voices and different interests. Ideally, it is about understanding differences, finding common ground and negotiating mutually acceptable solutions. It is about valuing alternative perspectives and thinking about things in new ways. If this is what public involvement should be about, the planning of public involvement should, perhaps, embrace similar values.

In most of our case studies, the planning of public involvement was a collaboration (see page 30). The people involved always had a common interest in public involvement, but this was typically driven by diverse values and by different ideas about what public involvement could and should achieve. But although different individuals wanted different things from their public involvement work, they did not necessarily have to do different things. Most of the aims of public involvement are complementary, such that any one method can deliver on several fronts at once.

The more people who got involved in the planning process, the broader the emergent vision of what public involvement could achieve. Broad visions not only helped to keep everyone on board, they also defined a wider range of potential outcomes for the chosen methods – though there could still be conflict about the priority of these outcomes.

Outcomes are what really matter

Whatever aims may be defined for public involvement initiatives, it is the outcomes which really matter.

North Lewisham began its public involvement work by bringing together a small group of key stakeholders from across the local health economy. The group spent time early on developing a strategy which brought together their wide-ranging concerns, including the quality of corporate decision-making, the needs of marginalised communities, equity of service provision, and the role of the voluntary and community sector in mediating public voices.

Although the strategy was not referred to much after it was finalised, it established a breadth of vision which valued everyone's role and kept everyone on board. Over time, the membership of the group changed as more people became involved. However, having established a broad vision at the outset, the changing membership sustained a discussion about the aims and impact of public involvement work without feeling that these issues had been settled. This helped the group to be both flexible in its understanding of what the work should achieve while also being vigilant about the actual impact of particular initiatives.

We haven't done anything except meet and talk, and I didn't want us to. I wanted us just to talk and to get some of the sort of basic ideas and concepts out on the table, and the fact that there might be differences in interest between the people around the table. And to get people to think in terms of the sort of spectrum of participation, and that they were already doing some of these things, and feeding that back to the PCG so that we're not starting from scratch. We don't need to be tokenistic: we can take our time to do things that are real, that are going to have a real impact on people's lives.

Lay member

Although there are many examples of public involvement work delivering very little, the potential is enormous. In effective public involvement, everyone stands to gain: lay participants, professionals, officers, community organisations and, in the longer term, the community and patient population.

Public involvement is therefore best pursued not only with a broad view of its potential outcomes but also with an openness and sensitivity to the diversity of actual outcomes.

The experience of public involvement is full of surprises (as well as disappointments). It is not a bad thing if people change their ideas about what an initiative can achieve as they go along if this means that they are valuing the emergent strengths of the work.

This does not mean that it is acceptable to 'muddle through' in the hope that something good will come of it all. Attention to the diversity of outcomes in practice should be part of a critical interest in achieving change. Furthermore, whatever the outcomes of particular initiatives, the people who get involved need to know what difference their input has made.

Harrow East & Kingsbury public involvement subgroup was charged with planning a patient survey to assess the quality of local diabetic care. They soon realised that this would be methodoogically impossible, given the diverse ethnic mix of this population. Instead, they organised a series of focus groups which evolved into on-going support groups. As well as being personally valuable for the participants who attended, the groups gave the specialist nurse who ran them lots of insight into ways in which local services could be improved. Although the PCG never got its assessment of quality, it did get an incremental process of service improvement.

Setting goals is still important

Developing a broad vision of public involvement work has its risks. All too easily, a general consensus about aims is not worked out in terms of specific goals. Without clear goals, methods can rapidly take over. One-off events often require great effort to organise, leaving people exhausted afterwards when their closer attention to impact may be needed. Similarly, standing mechanisms can take on a life of their own, diverting attention from the question of whether they are actually making any difference.

The broad aims which people define for public involvement can be very hard to translate into specific goals for specific initiatives. Complex changes in culture, subtle changes in organisational process, gradual changes in attitudes and behaviour – none of these are easy to specify, identify or evaluate. The identification of specific goals usually requires some kind of compromise along the long chain of impact and outcomes. For example, which of the following is an appropriate goal for a public consultation event?

- lots of people turning up to the event
- attendance by key PCG decision-makers
- critical discussion between public and professionals during the meeting
- the completion of a detailed report from the event
- PCG board members reading the report
- PCG board members discussing and approving the report
- specific changes to policy
- specific changes to professional practice
- improvements in the user experience of services
- improvements in patient health
- improvements in patient quality of life.

This is only one chain of events. There are others, for example, for the individuals who attend the initial event and for the community organisations represented at the event.

In our case studies, people involved in planning public involvement were always dealing with such cascades of 'outputs' and 'outcomes'. Inevitably, one person's outcome would often be another person's output – i.e. just a step along the way to what 'really' matters. There is no final way of deciding where to draw such lines. It is always important to set immediate goals (it matters that 100 people turn up rather than five) but this should not be at the expense of attention to impact beyond the initiative, method or role itself.

Delivering change is the hardest, and arguably most neglected, part of public involvement work (see Chapter 9). It is here that specific goals are difficult to set, not least because they are likely to be dependent on the public involvement process itself. Nonetheless, commitment at the outset to achieving identifiable changes in policy or practice is vital if critical reflection on internal impact is to take place after the event.

In our case studies, the importance of seeing public involvement through to real change was widely acknowledged, but regular, critical attention to the

I don't know what my expectations were. I tried not to have any, except that I feel it's all a little bit pointless if it doesn't make a difference, and I'm not yet entirely sure how or where it will. But it could be a way of making the service more responsive to patients.

Lay member

City & Hackney PCG was required to consult on its plans to become a primary care trust. Such requirements usually inspire consultations which aim solely to get over the hurdle and move on. Happily, the PCG approached the challenge with more imagination. It sought to turn the consultation into an opportunity to really listen to local people about their experience of local services and their concerns about community health. The aim was to build a shared vision of the new organisation and its priorities.

The process involved outreach by officers to dozens of local community group meetings, talking to people on their own turf and, as far as possible, on their own terms. This process helped to build trust and communication between the organisation and its local communities. It also produced a clear agenda for change for the new PCT.

The members of the PCG judged the consultation successful because of the number of groups attended, the quality of the debate and the diversity of the issues raised. However, the PCG did not have the capacity to take forward the results – it was a year before any action was taken. Although the board was right to value the success of the consultation in achieving its process goals, it did not pay the same critical attention to its internal goals. In part, this was because they could not be well-defined at the outset, as the agenda for change was to be the product of the consultation. And whereas the consultation had discrete process goals, the goals it defined were easily lost within the flood of organisational development goals the PCG had to tackle.

issue was rare. When people did try to grapple with what this meant in practice, they were easily frustrated by the difficulty of identifying any specific changes in an organisation that was changing all the time anyway.

What can public involvement deliver?

Public involvement is messy, open-ended, constantly renegotiated and always liable to get bogged down in methods precisely because different stakeholders have so many different ideas about what it can achieve.

There are lots of ways of categorising the aims which people identify for public involvement work (see over). The approach here does no more than give a flavour of the possibilities, but continues to make the link between aims and individual values and interests. Each of the following accounts is rooted in individual roles, responsibilities and commitments.

John, chief officer

John had a clear operational focus on getting the service to deliver. He knew that this could not be done in isolation – he needed the support of local agencies and local people. For John, the aims of public involvement were:

- to improve organisational decision-making
- to inform the development of more effective services and the better use of the resources available
- to gain public support for the PCG and its development plans.

Margaret, lay member

Margaret had lots of experience working with marginalised communities in the area and knew that the health service had to change radically if it was to address the needs of all of its local population adequately. She wanted everyone to be partners in the improvement of the health of local people. For Margaret, the aims of public involvement were:

- to enable local people to have a voice in local discussions about health improvement, and some control over their health and the health of their communities

In the public interest: developing a strategy for public participation in the NHS

NHS Executive, Institute of Health Services Management, NHS Confederation. Wetherby: Department of Heath, 1998.

This government-sponsored report was striking in the breadth of its vision. It presented a rationale for public involvement in the NHS which encompassed outcomes for the organisation, its users, local people and local communities. The following benefits were described:

Benefits to the NHS
- Restoration of public confidence
- Improved outcomes for individual patients
- More appropriate use of health services
- Potential for greater cost effectiveness
- Contribution to problem resolution
- Sharing responsibilities for health care with the public

Benefits to people
- Better outcomes of treatment and care
- An enhanced sense of self esteem and capacity to control their own lives
- A more satisfying experience of using health services
- More accessible, sensitive and responsive health services
- Improved health
- A greater sense of ownership of the NHS

Benefits to public health
- Reduction in health inequalities
- Improved health
- Greater understanding of the links between health and the circumstances in which people live their lives
- More healthy environmental, social and economic policies

Benefits to communities and to society as a whole
- Improved social cohesion
- A healthier democracy – reducing the democratic deficit
- A health service better able to meet the needs of its citizens
- More attention to cross-cutting policy issues and closer co-operation between agencies with a role to play in health improvement

- to change the culture of the health service from defensiveness and secrecy to openness and trust
- to improve local services through a close understanding of community needs, valuing all forms of local community intelligence.

Mark, health authority non-executive member on PCG board

Mark's role meant that he was involved in lots of strategic discussions about the future of the PCG and local health services. However, he was committed to public involvement at all levels of the institution's activity. For Mark, the aims of public involvement were:

- to secure the accountability of the institution and the proper use of public money
- to shape an agenda for community health improvement in partnership with the local community, based on community intelligence
- to ensure that all services and service developments were sensitive to user experience, needs and interests
- to encourage greater partnership with patients and carers in everyday professional practice.

Evan, patient participation group chair

Evan was a member of the PCG's public involvement working group, but his main role was as chair of a long-established patient participation group. For Evan, the aims of patient participation were:

- to inform and educate patients and carers about the practice, the role of the professionals based there and their own role in managing their health and the health of their families
- to improve the relationships between the professionals in the surgery and the patients and carers who attended
- to maximise communication between professionals and local people
- to build a sense of community around the surgery.

Susan, development manager

Susan was very focussed on the development of primary care services but knew her limitations and the limitations of health service professionals in

In my view, communication is the be all and end all. Because if we're all going our own ways and nobody is communicating with anybody else, sooner or later there is going to be an omission or crash isn't there, so I would seriously think that the point should be laboured. Good communication, let people know what you're doing, and consultation before action.

Patient participation group chair

Which champions, which people? Public and user involvement in health care as a technology of legitimation

Harrison S and Mort M. *Social Policy & Administration*. 1998; vol. 32 no.1: 60–70.

For all the potential of public involvement, in practice it can still be overwhelmed by institutional priorities. Harrison and Mort explored NHS use of health panels and user group relationships. The common feature of all their examples was the priority of managerial interests in shaping final outcomes. Of the panels, they noted that:

> *'Great care is taken by the authorities not to commit themselves to taking action on the results of the consultations. This is usually said to be because the views of 'the public' must be (later) balanced with other views.'*

Similarly, the user groups were manipulated within managerial 'strategic micropolitics':

> *'The simultaneous construction of user groups' legitimacy by the expression of positive views about them, and its deconstruction by reference to their unrepresentativeness and/or unsatisfactoriness as formal organisations, constitutes a device by which whatever stance officials might take in respect of user group preferences or involvement on particular issues could be justified.'*

The authors describe this organisational desire for legitimation through public involvement both as a means of deflecting the lack of democracy within the NHS and as a response to the loss of the hierarchy which gave local NHS organisations legitimacy prior to the 1990s health service reforms.

It would be impossible to paint such a bleak picture from our cases studies. Other than the policy shift from markets to partnership, a key difference is the individuals who acted as local 'champions' of public involvement. In the cases Harrison and Mort investigated, these were typically PR or communications officers. In our studies, PR officers either were not around (because primary care groups had such small executives) or were not involved. The champions were lay members, senior officers, and people from community health councils and voluntary organisations. The presence of more 'outsider' voices helped to ensure that critical attention was paid to outcomes beyond shoring up the interests of the organisation.

Nonetheless, power lay with the institutions. There was considerable frustration with the inability of primary care organisations to really grasp the lessons of public involvement. Public involvement initiatives *were* used to legitimate corporate decisions determined by professional interests. But, as long as there were outsider voices close to the heart of the primary care organisation, the organisational drive to legitimation was always in tension with the drive for real change.

general. For Susan, the aims of public involvement were:

- to ensure that the development of services was shaped by an understanding of local needs
- to challenge professional and policy assumptions about the best way of delivering services
- to provide on-going improvements in the quality and efficiency of service delivery.

Liz, community development worker

Liz worked with local community organisations, building networks, enabling joint working and supporting links with the PCG. She felt strongly that the PCG undervalued the insight which these organisations had into community needs and their potential in addressing these needs. For Liz, the aims of public involvement were:

- to increase the voluntary/community sector role in achieving health improvement in the area
- to ensure that PCG decision-making was responsive to the needs and interests of local people and local organisations
- to increase the capacity of community organisations to engage with and influence statutory bodies.

These examples illustrate the diversity of the possible aims of public involvement work. But they also reiterate the need for negotiation: it may be possible to pursue all these aims at once, but if there is no clarity about different interests, someone is likely to end up disappointed.

What we're seeking to achieve is to understand how people perceive the care that they are receiving, and so how perhaps the organisation of the care could be improved/enhanced – anything that's going to make their life easier, anything that's going to lead towards better health results – and just taking on board what the patients have got to say about these services, and seeking hopefully to bring about change if it is felt that things could change for the better.

Officer

Chapter six

Turning to others

KEY POINTS

Expertise in public involvement is likely to be dispersed across a health economy and so is maximised through collaboration.

Collaborative planning also increases the potential for cross-institutional learning from public involvement initiatives, as public perspectives do not respect institutional boundaries.

Existing public involvement mechanisms may offer relatively low-cost opportunities for primary care organisations to exploit.

The more substantial task of working in partnership requires much greater investment, particularly in time, effort and patience.

Primary care organisations almost always turn to others for help and support in the development of their public involvement work. However, the relationships they build are diverse. 'Partnership' is used to describe everything from occasional networking to collaborative work in the pursuit of shared goals. For those with the fullest commitment to partnership work, public involvement is itself part of the greater challenge of partnership: engaging with all local voices, inside and outside the institutions of a health economy.

This chapter describes some of these differences, exploring:

- the benefits of collaborative planning
- the value of sharing learning from public involvement
- the potential for exploiting existing practice
- the challenge of developing collaborative practice
- some of the practical difficulties involved.

Collaborative planning

Planning public involvement in collaboration with other local stakeholders has many potential benefits for primary care organisations. Primary care has not traditionally been the hottest spot for public involvement, so it makes sense for primary care organisations to turn to others to share experience, expertise, ideas and local knowledge – as well as values, commitment and enthusiasm. Conversations across the health economy also help to avert duplication of work and 'consultation fatigue' among local people.

In four of our case studies, the primary care organisation established some form of standing collaborative group to help give direction to their public involvement work. In every one of these groups there was representation from the local community health council and from the voluntary sector, with less universal representation from health authorities, local authorities, NHS trusts, tenants' groups and patient participation groups. The members of these groups had diverse interests, values and responsibilities. They included members and officers, frontline workers and chief executives, paid officers and patient representatives.

These groups were not joint investment groups – if money was discussed at all, it was only the primary care group's money on the agenda. However, they were opportunities for everyone to share and pursue their different but overlapping interests. Planning was therefore always a negotiation between different values, priorities and interests (see page 38).

The groups were places not only to share ideas and plan new work, but also to reflect on and improve current practice. At best, they were opportunities for shared learning about the practice of public involvement across the local health economy.

The two primary care organisations that did not set up working groups also turned to community health councils and the voluntary sector to plan their work. One had regular meetings with the community health council; the other relied on communication through operational relationships. Both, but particularly the latter, suffered from the lack of opportunities to reflect on practice, share experience and ideas, and build a common understanding of the value of the work.

There are a number of projects that have been around that have been making recommendations – community projects and self-help groups – that never actually influence policies because there's no mechanism for that to happen. It's actually a question of the PCG making itself aware of all those things and utilising that information and the intelligence that's out there. It's a two-way process really: it's about the PCG linking up with what already exists and what work has already been done, even if it's not in original form, and the second is to support more initiatives largely like that.

Officer

Sharing learning

Public views do not sit neatly within institutional boundaries. Consequently, learning from public involvement work is rarely relevant to only one organisation, unless the agenda is set very narrowly (see page 52). A process of shared learning from public involvement initiatives helps to ensure that public voices reach the places where change is possible.

Sharing learning can be remarkably difficult to achieve in practice. It is hard enough for primary care organisations to learn through their own public involvement work (see page 55), let alone through work which they have no stake in. Gaining such a stake is another benefit of planning in collaboration, though the learning from local public involvement has to go well beyond joint planning groups.

In only one of our case studies was an explicit attempt made to identify learning from existing public involvement work and actively use it within the organisation. Elsewhere, transmission of such learning relied on informal processes, particularly the participation in the primary care organisation (in any way) of individuals with local experience and knowledge.

Exploiting existing practice and opportunities

In all of our case studies, primary care organisations were keen to exploit existing opportunities rather than having to invest in setting up new ones from scratch. 'Exploit' is not used here in a derogatory way. It makes good sense to maximise the value of what already exists, but this may simply mean that primary care organisations make the most of existing resources for their own interests, rather than trying to identify and build on shared interests. This may involve the use of existing mechanisms to ask questions of relevance to primary care. Alternatively, it may simply mean having a presence at someone else's event or using a newsletter or forum for one-off communication and feedback.

This is all good practice, although some mechanisms of public involvement are more amenable to this

As part of their strategic development process, North Lewisham funded a short-term post with the aim of drawing together all local 'community intelligence' that had been gained through public involvement and community research work. This involved collating results from a wide variety of reports and talking in detail to local stakeholders with personal knowledge of the health needs of the community and experience of local consultation. The final report was substantial and gave the PCG a clear set of messages about community priorities. However, the process of getting these messages into the heart of the organisational development process was as difficult for this piece of work as it had been for all the reports which it drew on.

The public involvement subgroup in Harrow East & Kingsbury did not feel it had the capacity to develop its own methods of involvement, so looked to other local initiatives for help. The borough's citizens' panel was well-established and seemed an obvious route to gaining public views about health services, independent from their actual use. The group developed a survey about attitudes and use of local health services, which was duly distributed to members of the citizens' panel. The results proved to be very timely for the PCG members, but were of little relevance to the borough. The borough had not been a partner in its development and so had no stake in the results.

treatment than others. For example, a citizens' panel may be used by a variety of organisations for their own purposes but a coalition of community groups may not be happy in being treated as a 'sink' for consultation documents.

Developing collaborative practice

Collaborative practice in public involvement is still relatively uncommon. The health of a community may depend on the work of a multitude of organisations, but every organisation still has its own priorities and interests to pursue. Although the NHS has a duty of partnership, most practical experience is limited to collaborative planning and joint commissioning rather than collaborative practice. In primary care, experience of working with other organisations is particularly rare.

Working in partnership requires an understanding of mutual interests as well as clarity about different roles. Both of these can take time to negotiate and resolve. Partnerships are about building relationships of trust in which both partners invest for rewards beyond their independent potential (see over).

This investment need not be principally financial. Partnerships need time, effort, commitment and patience. In our case studies, the primary care organisations were hard pushed to find these resources for their public involvement work. Moving from the open discussions of collaborative planning to the detailed work of collaborative practice was not easy.

A key problem in the case studies was the transience of the primary care groups themselves. It is hard to build working relationships when your own future is in serious doubt. This perennial problem for the health service continues to create real frustration among all its potential partners in local communities.

Some practical difficulties

Negotiating across diverse interests. This is what partnership, and public involvement, is all about. But it remains one of the trickiest tasks, requiring a combination of sensitivity and leadership – valuing differences while also building a degree of consensus.

What we've been doing is putting together a document, which isn't so much a strategy but just details what everybody is doing. So we found out about things that the local authority does on a regular basis but also a Tenants' Survey, into which we could maybe put questions periodically. So instead of us doing our own surveys and risking people just chucking it in the bin because they only had one the day before, we are trying to work co-operatively across organisations.

Lay member

In Hayes & Harlington, the community health council (CHC) had established a close working relationship with local primary care professionals prior to the creation of the PCG. This meant that the CHC was in a good position to support the development of the new PCG's public involvement work, which it did by funding and running a standing public panel. The lay members participated in the panel meetings and reported back to the PCG board, and other officers and members also regularly attended. For the PCG, it was a valuable public sounding board. For the CHC, it provided useful insight into both institutional and public priorities. Although there were sometimes tensions between the two organisations about the group's agenda, it proved to be a fruitful partnership for both.

In City & Hackney, the chair of the public involvement subgroup was approached by the chair of the local tenants convention to discuss joint working. The convention appeared to offer a ready-made route for two-way consultation with local people. Both parties recognised that this should be a relationship, not just another place to send documents for consultation. This required that members or officers of the PCG spend time going to the meetings and engaging with the convention on its own terms. Unfortunately, no-one had the time to do this adequately. Despite the best of intentions to build sustainable relationships across the local health economy, the potential of the convention for the PCG was lost.

Making partnerships work. A practical guide for the public, private, voluntary and community sectors.

Wilson A and Charlton K. York: Joseph Rowntree Foundation, 1997.

This book offers a practical approach to working in partnership, drawing on research into 12 cross-sector partnerships in the UK. The authors describe the drive for partnership as being intimately linked with the drive for public involvement:

> 'The notion of partnership fits in with emerging concepts of communitarianism and a stakeholder society… In many areas – for example education, health care and crime prevention – people are no longer prepared to sit back and let "the authorities" dictate what is done, when, and how. Individuals and organisations from all sectors are increasingly demanding a voice in defining and implementing the most appropriate responses to many of the challenges facing society.'

A five-stage model for partnership management is described:

- The partners come together through the mutual recognition of a common need, or in a joint effort to obtain public funds.
- Through a process of dialogue and discussion, the partners establish the common ground and work towards agreeing a vision and mission statement for the initiative.
- The formal framework and organisational structure of the partnership is designed and put in place.
- The partnership delivers to its action plan, whether this be service provision or some other function.
- Where appropriate, the partners plan their exit strategy. This involves developing a new set of goals for the survival and continuation of the work of the initiative in some form.

This model is a useful reminder of the extent of corporate commitment and resources required for serious engagement in collaborative work. No such partnerships existed in our cases studies. Strategic partnership work was beginning within the primary care organisations, but the focus of the work was typically on the core service concerns of the organisation, not the relatively marginal issue of public involvement.

Nonetheless, these strategic partnerships all embraced the voluntary sector and were committed to public involvement. They may provide opportunities in the future for collaborative approaches to the design and implementation of public involvement work as a whole. However, care is needed to ensure that the formal arrangements required when organisations share resources and responsibilities enable, rather than inhibit, openness and creativity in public involvement work.

Meetings all too easily slide into unfocussed discussions; but with too strong a chair, participants can feel undervalued or alienated.

Talk and action. Skill is also required in getting the balance right between the consensus-building discussion and the detail of implementation. If not enough time is spent sharing ideas and interests, public involvement initiatives may run their course without connections being made to anyone else's work and influence in the health economy. Too little action, and disillusion and frustration soon set in. The more people there are involved in the discussion, the more difficult it can be to make choices about where to act, because this involves also deciding where not to act. Making choices between the various interests represented in any partnership forum is never easy.

Marginalisation. Bringing people together to develop collaborative approaches to public involvement work ought to reduce the risk or marginalisation. However, the creation of any new institution – such as a working group or partnership forum – always runs the risk of marginalising the issue from the existing institutions. Such groups have to be well-connected with the rest of the business of the organisation if they are to be effective in ensuring that such work brings about change.

Confusion of functions. Because the practice of partnership is so similar to the practice of public involvement, partnership meetings about planning public involvement can easily be mistaken for public involvement events in themselves. It may be difficult for participants from outside the organisation, including voluntary sector representatives, to stick rigorously to the public involvement planning agenda if they have few other opportunities to talk to members and officers. In practice, it can be difficult to keep these functions apart. In our case studies, all four of the partnership groups for planning public involvement were also used by participants as opportunities to raise other policy and practice issues with the members and officers of the primary care organisations concerned. It is therefore important to regularly review the terms of reference of such groups, so that members' perceptions of what they are for are not too divergent.

Public involvement lends itself to a sense of freedom, a sense of experiment, exploring other ways of doing things. But it's still mostly about plugging in to all the main players and networking out there with what's already happening. It has been very little to do with innovation, just slogging through the corridors, going to see this one and that one and making sure he is happy and she is happy. It's about diplomacy. And I think it's less about personal involvement. You get the occasional individuals that will come and share and want to make a difference, but it's about working with the big players really at the moment.

Officer

Chapter seven

Corporate essentials?

KEY POINTS

Public involvement work in primary care organisations requires a minimum of individual enthusiasm and the support of a senior officer. With these, something is always achievable, whatever the corporate obstacles.

Commitment at board level is important, but is no guarantee that anything will happen in practice. It may be crucial to long-term culture change, but will only grow through experience.

Leadership may come from members, officers or even stakeholders outside the organisation.

Public involvement initiatives need not be high cost but organisations have to invest in internal follow-through if they are to learn from public voices.

Strategies for public involvement need to be flexible if they are to be as valuable in their implementation as they are in their development and approval.

What are the key ingredients which a primary care organisation needs to enable it to undertake public involvement work?

This chapter gives a qualified answer to this question. It is impossible to be prescriptive about what every primary care organisation needs. In each of our case studies, certain 'essentials' were lacking or in short supply, but in each case progress was made. Progress depended, in part, on the skill of local stakeholders in playing to their strengths and working around their weaknesses.

Each of the following was widely *perceived* to be essential:

- commitment
- leadership
- resources
- strategies.

The importance of each proved to be variable in practice, depending on how local people responded to local circumstances.

Corporate commitment

The actions of primary care organisations are not determined entirely by the decision-makers on the board, but depend on the power, persuasiveness and influence of all the people who have a stake in the organisation. So although the attitudes and priorities of board members are important, they are not critical to everything that a primary care organisation tries to do.

As long as there are some people within the organisation with personal commitment to public involvement, there are usually ways and means of making progress. Perhaps the only other essential is the support of a senior officer, ideally the chief officer. Without commitment among the people actually doing the work, other priorities inevitably push public involvement out of the corporate in-tray.

In our case studies, board commitment to public involvement was widely perceived to be important, but it did not guarantee that anything actually happened. It is easy enough for members to sign up to the principle but pay little attention to the practice. In such circumstances, public involvement work may simply be ignored. This may be more harmful than explicit opposition among members, which at least challenges individual advocates to make the case for public involvement and demonstrate its value.

Corporate commitment may be essential to the long-term process of changing organisational culture to be open and responsive to user and public voices. But in the short and medium term, what matters is that the key advocates of the work are willing to exploit enthusiasm where they find it and to work around (or bring round) people who show doubt, resistance or neglect. Corporate attitudes are only likely to change through experience.

In every one of our case studies, lay members played a role in keeping public involvement on the corporate agenda, though some were more effective in building support across (and beyond) the organisation than others. Other corporate champions included chief officers, community health council representatives and nurse members.

In Dagenham, GP board members were not interested in public involvement and did not value the contribution of the lay member. Although this was a very difficult experience for the lay member, she was deeply committed to listening to community voices and enlisted the support of other members and the chief officer to press her cause. The members of the public involvement subgroup, who each brought great personal enthusiasm, recognised that board attitudes were part of a wider failure by local primary care professionals to treat their users as partners. Consequently, they managed to secure funding for a training programme in patient partnership for all local primary care professionals.

In City & Hackney, all board members accepted the value of public involvement and welcomed the lay member in corporate debates. They also funded substantial outreach work with local community groups. However, the PCG's public involvement work rarely challenged their own practice or decision making. It remained one of the things to be done, but not something that they had to pay much attention to on a packed organisational development agenda.

If change is sought among the constituent practices of a primary care organisation rather than in its corporate heart, local commitment is also needed. Primary health care teams are small organisations in themselves. If there is no existing enthusiasm within them for public involvement, progress is likely to be very slow. In three of our case studies, significant efforts were made by the primary care organisation to develop public involvement work at practice level and, in each, the need to invest in winning the professionals over was underestimated. Although in each of these three cases there were 'champions' of public involvement among their frontline professionals, the fragmentation of primary care services meant that the influence of these individuals on their peers across the local area was minimal.

Corporate leadership

Keeping something on the agenda is not the same as making it happen. Leadership is here taken to mean the active process of ensuring that commitment is realised in action.

Lay members may have been obvious corporate choices to lead public involvement but there was concern in some PCGs that this was a marginalizing tactic, both for lay members and for public involvement. There was a strong case that lay members ought to be concerned with all the business of the organisation, and public involvement ought to be the responsibility of all the members of the board. But, again, practice was more complex than these neat solutions. Leadership had to fall to individuals. In all our case studies, lay members played an important role in promoting public involvement, regardless of whether they were formally delegated this role or not.

The key strength of lay member leadership was their insider connections. As members of the organisation, lay members could bring user and public perspectives to all sorts of internal decision-making – board meetings, subgroup meetings and day-to-day discussions. They could bridge the interests of outsiders and insiders. But lay member leadership was compromised if the individual did not have experience or understanding of the broader aspects of public involvement. Under these circumstances, lay

In Central Croydon, the link person scheme required that all local practices should support an individual from the practice in communicating the interests of the practice population to the PCG (and vice versa). But the PCG recruited the link patients directly and in some cases the practice staff were unaware that they had a link patient. Little effort was put into getting the support and interest of the practice staff before the scheme was set up. Consequently, many of the link people felt isolated and ignored by the professionals in their practices.

In Dagenham, the public involvement subgroup decided to encourage local GPs to follow the example of the one thriving patient participation group in the area. The chair of the PPG and the lay member wrote to practices and offered to go and talk issues through with interested GPs. Although this process began, it proved to be too great a task for their combined resources. Sustained support was needed to turn sceptical GPs into enthusiasts for patient participation.

In Hayes & Harlington, the two lay members were delegated the responsibility of leading public involvement work for the PCG. However, they were both relatively inexperienced in this work, and relied on the chief executive for direction, and the community health council for support and guidance. The community health council's chief officer had played an important role in shaping the form of the PCG's public involvement work and continued to be influential. Leadership was, in practice, distributed between these four stakeholders – each playing a key role in ensuring the progress of the public involvement work. In time, the lay members gained greater confidence in their roles. Their close involvement with the subgroups helped to ensure that all the officers and members were exposed to public views, thereby building corporate ownership of the public involvement work.

members had to turn to others for help. Leadership in practice was often a shared process.

The other formal leaders of the primary care organisations, chairs and chief officers, tended to be overwhelmed by the rest of the organisational agenda and could devote little time to public involvement. However, this was not entirely an obstacle. People who have an intimate understanding of the whole organisation's business may be best placed to identify where public involvement work can be useful in furthering the organisation's interests and work. Effective leadership at this level need not demand a lot of time if it is principally concerned with identifying and promoting these opportunities.

In our case studies, board chairs played minor roles (if any) in public involvement leadership, although the majority did ensure that the public meetings were properly open to, and respectful of, public views. They were all GPs with little experience of lay involvement in professional interests. However the chief officers did play important roles. They were all supportive of public involvement and ensured that public involvement initiatives were taken seriously within their organisations. Their support was necessary to the people who were developing the public involvement work and their leadership was particularly important at those junctures when the messages from public involvement had to be grasped by the organisation.

Leadership also came from outside. Where local partnerships were strong, certain voluntary sector and community health council officers played crucial roles not only in supporting but also in defining NHS public involvement work.

Corporate resources

Despite the prominence given to public involvement in policy, both nationally and locally, it remains chronically under-funded. Where money is forthcoming, it is likely to be for specific pieces of work rather than for sustained organisational support, making it hard to develop approaches to public involvement that systematically connect patient, carer and public voices with organisational interests.

Public involvement need not depend on large pots of new money. It may take a lot of money to run a

In North Lewisham, the lay member chaired the working group that planned the PCG's public involvement work – a leadership role that he was completely comfortable with. However, when he ceased to be the lay member, the group's chair was eventually taken by the director of a local voluntary organisation. The group had by this time become much bigger and was focussed on networking and building a shared vision rather than detailed planning. It was therefore possible for someone outside the organisation to play a strategic leadership role for the PCG's public involvement work while implementation of PCG initiatives was left to individual officers. However, the dispersal of the leadership role across a number of initiatives meant that it was harder to ensure that their value as a whole was maximised for the organisation.

I would like to see some PCG staff time devoted to the area of public involvement, because I think that's crucial. You know, however good I may or may not be, I am part-time, I have a full-time job, so I can't devote the time. I would like to see someone at staff level to move this whole agenda forward. Someone who can get on to it and do things more promptly and spend time making contacts and designing things and so forth. Now whether that's realistic with the limited resources we have, I don't know.

Lay member

citizens' jury or a community research project, but working in an open and inclusive way with local community stakeholders simply requires a bit of time from everyone (though 'everyone' may need training and support to use this time effectively). Thinking of involvement work as a set of (expensive) methods can undervalue approaches to involvement which are focussed on relationships and on-going dialogue.

Nonetheless, every relationship and every dialogue has to be supported and sustained. Every method of involvement has to connect to an internal process of learning. Whatever the costs of specific involvement projects, there has to be internal investment to ensure that user and public voices contribute to organisational learning and change.

In our case studies, very little investment was made either in the front-end involvement work or the internal process of change. There were too many priorities, too much to do, and too few resources to match. In only one of the primary care organisations was there an officer with some clearly dedicated officer time for public involvement. This meant that public involvement work was almost always an extra demand on the time of officers who had more pressing things to attend to. Inevitably, this meant that their focus was on getting something done rather than working with the organisation to learn from what was done.

In general, greater resources are also needed to reach further into the local population, to engage with the diversity of local communities and grapple with health issues on other people's terms. This is where existing community resources come into their own. The community resources available to a primary care organisation may be huge. By tapping into local networks and communicating though existing channels, primary care organisations can begin a process of community engagement at relatively low cost. However, the longer-term process of working in partnership with local communities requires investment in those communities. Supporting the development of community infrastructure is integral to the core primary care goal of health improvement, but also enables an ever-wider range of people to contribute to NHS policy and decision-making.

Hayes & Harlington developed a programme of public involvement at relatively low cost. This was achieved by emphasising the role of the lay members and drawing on the support of the community health council. The lay members were active on most of the PCG subgroups, to which they brought their own views as lay people, the views of members of the public panel (run and funded by the CHC) and the views of members of local groups whom they visited. Although there was a limit to the capacity of the two lay members, it was an efficient approach because they were engaged in the internal discussion and decision-making as well as doing the outreach and the listening.

Using a small commissioning budget and several one-off grants, North Lewisham supported a broad programme of public involvement work, including practice-based needs assessment, special consultation days and extensive voluntary sector partnership work. However, there was a perceived failure to ensure that all this work added up to a process of change. Resources were needed, and eventually identified, for someone to work within the organisation to make sure that all local user and public voices were carried through to changes in policy and practice.

In terms of resources, part of my brief is to look at how we can link up with the local authorities around their consultation and communication strategy. They've got community involvement teams, they've got PR in place, and I think the other resource is tapping into regeneration initiatives. In terms of reaching out to groups and making people aware, then there's opportunities to advertise, make links, make people aware of what the PCG is doing. So there are all kinds of resources.

Officer

Corporate strategies

Strategies, and the development of strategies, serve a number of purposes.

The process of putting a public involvement strategy together enables people to share their values and interests, reflect on local practice and negotiate shared goals. The presentation of the completed strategy to the board is a defining moment of corporate commitment to public involvement. Once agreed, the strategy may be used to shape practice, monitor implementation and assess progress. However, it may just be forgotten.

These three core functions are all valid. If a strategy does get quietly forgotten after it has been agreed, this does not mean that its development has been in vain.

In our six case studies, only three of the primary care organisations produced public involvement strategies. For one, the development of the strategy was a valuable process for the key stakeholders concerned, enabling them to share ideas and develop a common sense of purpose and priorities. Although it was rarely referred to after its approval, it established a clear direction of travel. In the other two case studies, strategies were put together fairly quickly and did little more than describe existing practice. They were useful principally to ensure, or shore up, the commitment of the board to public involvement.

The failure to use strategies as critical documents for on-going practice reflects the general problems of planning in the health service and the particular difficulties of developing public involvement with minimal resources. In every case study, the people leading the work had to make the most of what they had in a rapidly changing policy environment. This meant exploiting existing practice and seizing opportunities when they arose. For some, sustaining any kind of public involvement work was an achievement, given the demands of the development agenda (although the development agenda also created new opportunities).

Not everyone was happy with this state of affairs. But there was little regret about the lack of strategy.

I think the problem that we're going to have is around building up too much expectation and not being able to meet them. Do we have the resources to support real community involvement and sustain change from the messages that we get back? I get quite excited about it because I think that there is some scope for us to do some real work with local people. But then I worry because we're still part of the bureaucracy of the NHS: we're still governed by financial restraints.

Chief officer

Concern was focussed more on the problems of achieving change through public involvement than lack of strategic documents. Strategies were not felt to be the answer to this problem, not least because other strategic documents, such as Health Improvement Programmes, were also felt to have a tenuous relationship to changes in practice.

There is clearly a strong case for developing public involvement strategies that are useful after they have been agreed: with nothing to give direction to new initiatives or monitor progress against, eclectic approaches can just become arbitrary approaches. However, public involvement is a messy business (see page 20), so any strategy must also be flexible enough to value all the outcomes of public involvement work and pick up on the ever-changing strengths of the local context.

The public involvement group has been set up and I chair it, but my perception is that the board think that that is being sorted out. What they don't realise is that I, personally, am finding it very difficult to know exactly what it means to come up with a strategy for public involvement, which is what I and the group are supposed to be doing. I feel it has been left to me and the group with perhaps insufficient terms of reference. The overall remit was to come up with a public involvement strategy, and only a week or two back have I ever seen such a document as a PCG Public Involvement Strategy, so I am really struggling to know the shape of what we are supposed to be working with.

Lay member

Chapter eight

Who – and whose agenda?

KEY POINTS

Distinctions between patients, carers, citizens and communities do not always identify different people, but rather the range of interests which public involvement seeks to address.

The diversity of local populations always presents difficult choices for public involvement work, particularly between targeting strong or excluded voices.

As well as targeted interventions, the enablement of excluded voices requires changes in professional attitudes, consistent attention to equal opportunities and investment in community infrastructure.

People who have gained stronger voices through the voluntary sector or institutional roles should be valued, not dismissed as 'inauthentic'.

In any public involvement, a bridge has to be built between institutional and public interests. Both have to be taken seriously for dialogue to succeed.

A primary care organisation has a responsibility for the health of its entire population. The question of whom to target for public involvement can therefore be daunting. At worst, concerns about equity and representation can inhibit people from doing anything at all. Yet there are plenty of ready opportunities – primary care organisations have easy access both to patient populations and to voluntary/community sector networks. Finding people to involve ought not to be a major problem in itself, though some communities inevitably present greater challenges than others.

This chapter explores some of the choices that are made by primary care organisations in the process of identifying and recruiting the 'public' to involve. It also explores a closely related issue: who sets the agenda. This chapter explores:

- basic population distinctions for NHS organisations
- addressing the diversity of local populations
- the problems created by perceptions of 'special interests'

- the problems created by anxieties about representation
- the bridge between organisational and public agendas.

Basic distinctions

For NHS organisations, a useful way of cutting the population cake is between patients, carers and the public. This is helpful because it identifies key differences in interests:

- Patients are users of services and so have an interest in the quality and delivery of those services.
- Informal carers have an interest both as providers and as users of health and social care.
- The public – local citizens – have an interest in the use of local resources and the impact of policy on local communities.

These distinctions are important for primary care organisations because of their responsibility for the health of the whole population, not just users of primary care. A focus solely on the GP patient population will not address this responsibility in full, though it may be a reasonable place to start.

These distinctions are not, however, between people but between interests – every patient is also a citizen, and every citizen is likely to be a patient or carer at some point. The model is a useful reminder of the range of interests that primary care organisations should address, but is not a clear signpost to specific groups to involve. In our case studies, primary care organisations recruited patients who were then involved in discussions about the health of the whole community, and citizens who were asked about their experience as patients and carers. Furthermore, users who achieve a collective voice to press for changes in service delivery are using the tool of citizenship to achieve their goals (see over).

The overwhelming interest of the public involvement subgroup in Harrow East & Kingsbury was their users' experience, but they chose to use the borough's citizens' panel for a health questionnaire. However, the focus of the questions was entirely on the panel members' knowledge and experience of health services. For the group, the strength of the method lay in its independence from a particular health service context, minimising the risk of respondents giving answers they feel their professional providers expect of them.

In Hayes & Harlington, a 'public' panel was recruited by the community health council, but to be a member of this panel you had to be registered as a patient with a local GP. The members of the panel were quite happy to discuss both 'patient' and 'public' issues – they were as comfortable talking about the development plans for local GP practices as they were discussing the public health priorities of the Health Improvement Programme.

In North Lewisham, community research to inform the development of a local GP practice included interviews with people recruited in the practice waiting rooms and interviews with people recruited on the street. The questions were the same, exploring experience of health services and broader factors affecting participants' health. Although many of the people on the street were also patients in the local practice, their answers, overall, were more critical of the health service and more focussed on social and environmental aspects of health. This illustrates the impact of context on individual perceptions: people will answer questions in more of a 'patient role' when they are asked them in a clinical rather than social context (and when illness is on their minds).

Users as citizens: collective action and the local governance of welfare

Barnes M. *Social Policy & Administration* 1999; vol. 33 no.1: 73–90.

Reflecting on both the history of the user movement and on evidence from a study of mental health user groups, Barnes explores the tensions between the interests of user groups and the interests of a state which is ever more keen to involve users in its decision-making.

It can be difficult for people within statutory organisations to value users as citizens. For citizenship is not simply about giving views but about changing things – and this almost always requires collective action. User organisations enable individuals to share collective experience, gain collective knowledge and achieve a collective voice. Having gained a collective voice, user organisations are unlikely to want only to help providers improve their services. They will also want to challenge their assumptions, question their priorities and call them to account. All of which can be fairly uncomfortable for providers and can prompt strategies to dismiss the collective voice in favour of the individual user.

The challenges experienced by professionals are matched by the threat of co-option experienced by user groups. In becoming part of the process of governance, such groups have to learn to work with institutional agendas as well as to question them. This is a tricky balance for all concerned. The process is often painful, but fruitful.

> 'User participation within systems of decision-making is enabled and supported by separate organization – users are often more effective participants if they have the support of others and can link into shared and common experiences, rather than speak solely from personal experience. Whilst participation carries the dangers of incorporation, there is also evidence of transformation taking place both in the processes of governance and the service models emerging between users and producers.'

Community and participation for general practice: perceptions of general practitioners and community nurses.

Brown I. *Social Science and Medicine*, 1994; vol. 39 no. 3: 335–344.

Brown explores the meanings of 'community' and 'participation' in general practice in inner Sheffield. Community was variously understood in terms of the local area, the practice population, ethnic differences and shared medical and social interests. A key tension emerged between individual and collective understandings:

> *'Taking community as locality or groups with shared interests as the organisational basis of community conflicted for some interviewees with the purpose and scope of general practice. For some, general practice is oriented to individual and practice population care rather than community in any other sense.'*

Participation was also understood on an individual-collective continuum, ranging from individual consumer choices to group empowerment.

Overall, Brown notes the dominance of individualism in general practice perspectives and the lack of a collective or communitarian ethic in its organisation. Although practice lists offer a basis of involvement work with users, a focus on shared medical and social needs could result in a community only being defined medically:

> *'It is surely important that people define their own communities and that organisations are flexible enough to interact with a plurality of communities whilst also prioritising those with greatest needs.'*

Since Brown's paper was published, primary care organisations have emerged, offering new perspectives on community, shaped by the core commitment to the health improvement of the local population. In our case studies, the result was a range of new interpretations of the tension between individualist and collective understandings of community.

In the context of public involvement work, only one of the primary care organisations completely ignored practice populations in favour of an understanding of community based on local demography: deprivation, ethnicity, locality. In the other five, practice populations always had some community value, but always as part of wider, more complex communities. The potential for involving people through practices was recognised but the interests of these participants were always assumed to be greater than their interests as practice users. Practice populations were never merely an 'administrative detail' because there was always potential for collective interests to be expressed within them, but such interests spilled beyond the immediate concerns of the practice staff – into the broader community concerns of the primary care organisation.

Addressing diversity

When faced with diverse populations, multiple communities, and complex patterns of illness and disability, it is not surprising that people embarking on public involvement work often feel overwhelmed. Commitment to equity in service provision can mean that choices about whom to engage in public involvement are difficult to make.

This should not become a stumbling block. Equity should be a goal which public involvement work serves, not a principle which undermines the confidence of a primary care organisation to undertake public involvement.

In our case studies, the need to listen to all local voices was always acknowledged, but in every case choices were made about who to prioritise for involvement work. These choices reflected both individual and corporate priorities. They can be understood in terms of the relative priority given to the following characteristics of both communities and individuals:

- extent of exclusion from services
- extent of exclusion from voice
- extent of health/healthcare need.

People who are excluded from services are, by definition, the hardest group for service providers to reach. They will also be excluded from having a voice in services and may well have significant health needs. Asylum seekers, homeless people, drug users, certain ethnic minorities and people dealing with isolation, extreme poverty, disability or mental health problems may all fall within this category. Public involvement work here is particularly challenging because of the difficulties in reaching the population and the complexity of the problems involved – many of which the primary care organisation may not be in a position to address. It is here that partnership approaches are likely to be most valuable.

People who are excluded from having a voice in health services include those who are excluded from services and those who are highly dependent on services. Those whose health care needs are such that they are very reliant on services, but also very vulnerable to changes in services, may be the least

City & Hackney had a particularly diverse population, characterised by large ethnic minority communities and high levels of poverty. The PCG knew that many local people were not registered with GPs and had little or no contact with primary and community health services. The PCG used the PCT consultation process as an opportunity to reach out to some of these people: going to dozens of local community groups to speak to people on their own turf about how the future of local services could better address their needs. Inevitably, there were many people with no connections to such groups, but this was a necessary first step towards a wider engagement with the local community.

Members of Dagenham's public involvement subgroup were very aware of the failures of the health service to give local people any voice in decisions about their services. The lay member's considerable experience in the local carers' association had exposed her to the powerlessness of highly dependent people in the face of the bureaucracy of the NHS. The research study into the voices of vulnerable people in the area was the result: a qualitative exploration of the experience of highly dependent patients and carers. The independent researcher commissioned to undertake the study noted that the methodological challenges of interviewing vulnerable people were considerable. What she heard was powerful, but it took time to build the confidence of the participants to speak their minds about the services they relied on – a process which could be exhausting for the participants.

confident in expressing their concerns to service providers. People with disabilities or chronic illness, housebound people, older people and carers may feel nervous about the impact of any criticism they make. Third party involvement may be necessary to engage with the voices of dependent or vulnerable users.

Professional assumptions have always played a role in excluding people from voice. Children and young people, people with mental health problems, older people, people with learning difficulties – all have been dismissed as incapable of articulating their own interests. This is a form of exclusion from voice which no NHS organisation can ignore.

Finally, there are all the obstacles which routinely exclude people from voice – language differences; difficulties with vision, speech and hearing; mobility problems; caring responsibilities, etc. Consideration of the basics of equal opportunities in public involvement work is still far from routine.

A variety of strategies were employed in our case studies to address these issues. They usually involved either trying to engage with people on their own turf – in their homes or community groups – or trying to provide the necessary support, such as interpreters, to overcome the obstacles excluding them from participation. Important though these strategies were, they did little to empower excluded voices – a process which requires considerably more investment in community infrastructure (see right).

People who have high health needs are an obvious and common target for public involvement work in primary care. Such work is often focussed on people who are users of services and willing to talk about their experience, i.e. those who are not excluded in the ways described above. The value of targeting confident service users is the wealth of immediately relevant information generated for providers. This information is likely to have a very direct bearing on the strategic and operational concerns of primary care organisations and so stands a good chance of achieving impact.

With limited resources for public involvement, primary care organisations have to be skilful in using them in targeted ways which bring about real change.

If we're doing a straightforward consultation process then we won't reach marginalised groups. But I think there are community groups and other groups out there who are working with those communities and that's why I think we need to support community development with those. We need to strengthen what's already out there. We have to look to where people are already doing work. There's a whole range of different groups in the community and voluntary sector that are working with these communities and that's why it's important that the PCG works with those because it can't do it on its own.

Officer

Harrow East & Kingsbury developed a successful programme of seminars and support groups for diabetics in the area. By focussing on a patient group with high needs, they had ready access to the population they wanted to involve. However, this population included a high proportion of South Asian patients, many of whom were not confident English speakers. Consequently, separate groups were run in Gujerati and Punjabi. An initial focus on high demand enabled the PCG to address problems of excluded voices with relative ease.

Public participation and marginalized groups: the community development model

O'Keefe E and Hogg C. *Health Expectations* 1999; vol. 2: 245–254.

O'Keefe and Hogg describe a programme of involvement work with housebound people which focussed on building confidence among its users through membership of an emergent community infrastructure.

The authors identify the following key features of the project:

- Building trust through personal contact prior to collective meetings.
- Sustaining relationships over the length of time necessary for collective voices to bring about change.
- Delivering benefits for members both as consumers (improvements in services) and citizens (shared learning and action).
- The independence of the programme from statutory providers, thereby minimising members' fears that voicing concerns could risk the services they depended on.

In our case studies, most of the involvement initiatives with marginalized groups were time-limited and could not begin to address the underlying development needs.

Community development featured in only one case study: North Lewisham. There were two distinct initiatives. A worker was funded to network with local community groups, building on their shared interests and supporting their involvement with the NHS. Also, a voluntary organisation worked in GP practices to identify and address the community health needs of patients and carers. The director of this organisation played an effective intermediary role, lobbying the GPs and the local statutory agencies to respond to these community needs. Both of these approaches helped to reduce the isolation of the primary care group and bring it into closer and wider contact with its local population.

O'Keefe and Hogg claim that *'public involvement needs to start from a users' perspective rather than from the point of view of the agenda of the statutory bodies'*, not least because members of the project had complex concerns which were not confined to health services. Yet the staff and members of the project had to work hard to ensure that their collective voices were taken seriously and acted on by local providers.

In our case studies, public involvement work rarely started from a user or public perspective. It started in many different places (at the same time) but always ended up as a negotiation between institutional and public voices. The community development initiatives strengthened the public voices in this negotiation but did not, as far as the primary care group was concerned, give them priority.

In making choices about whom to involve, they have to consider the relative costs and benefits of targeting both strong and excluded voices. Confident users may deliver the quickest (and cheapest) results, but the needs of excluded communities and individuals are likely to be much more acute.

Special interests

The question of who to involve is often complicated by a desire to reach 'real' patients and local people, rather than the familiar voices of local institutional and voluntary sector representatives. The voice of 'Jo Bloggs', the man or woman on the street with no special interests, is considered to be more authentic than the voices of the 'usual suspects'.

These distinctions are spurious and unhelpful. For a start, Jo Bloggs does not exist – everyone has special interests in their own health and the health of their families and communities. Public involvement work is about bringing different interests together, valuing them and finding the connections between them. This is what happens in the internal dialogue of the NHS, between professional interests, all the time. Suspicion of the interests of NHS outsiders only helps to keep them as outsiders.

In our case studies, the voluntary sector was never systematically excluded from public involvement work. However, there were differences in how voluntary sector organisations were valued. In some primary care organisations, they were treated as obvious partners, integral to the public involvement process. Elsewhere, they were treated as a resource for getting to public voices, rather than as a valuable voice in themselves.

A distinction between unproblematic individual interests and the 'special' interests of organisations has serious consequences for the former as well as the latter. For it indicates to individuals that if they seek to gain greater collective power and a stronger stake in the internal workings of the NHS, they will be treated less seriously by those on the inside. Even the casual dismissal of the 'usual suspects' can contribute to this.

Representation

'The usual suspects' may also be dismissed because they are 'not representative'. Anxiety about

I think that we need to involve our local community groups in all of this. A lot of the local groups have come out of community concerns and are people who are part of the community themselves and who have created organisations from that starting point. There is a received wisdom which you get waves of sometimes. A mindset that community groups are provider agencies with their hand out and that they will do what they need to in order to keep their organisation going. And there's this sort of assumption of a conflict of interest which comes out of the purchaser/provider split. We haven't had the level of political conversation to address this, and I'm hoping we can find a way to do it but we never have that depth of conversation anyway.

Lay member

representation can seriously inhibit public involvement work. A choice about who to involve necessarily means choosing who not to involve – and such a choice means that the approach must be unrepresentative. Better, then, not to make the choice at all.

The argument is ludicrous when presented like this, but it is not uncommon. In this form, the problem lies with the dominance of a quantitative research model in which any process of 'finding things out' has to be statistically representative if it is to be valid. As primary care organisations are run largely by clinical professionals, familiar with quantitative clinical research, these values are often expressed, despite the fact that professional decision-making both in the consulting room and in the board room is informed by a great deal more then statistically robust data.

Public involvement is not research. Research may be part of an approach to public involvement, but public involvement should not be judged overall with the values of research. In three of our case studies, significant pieces of research were undertaken as part of their public involvement work. However, in each case, the central and critical part of the public involvement process took place after the completion of the research: i.e. the communication of the results to the key decision-makers. Public involvement is, above all, about communication and dialogue, rather than simply finding things out.

Representation is also understood, and exploited, politically. According to the original NHSE guidance, lay members on PCG boards had to represent the interests of local communities. This was a red rag to various bulls: how could a single individual, appointed and not elected, with very limited time to engage with local people and bearing the responsibilities of the organisation 'represent' anyone other than themselves?

Inasmuch as this was used as an argument to undermine the authority of lay members, it was deeply unfair. After all, professional members did not have to justify their own representative role. In practice, every member of a PCG board had to find a balance between speaking for themselves and speaking for others. People who are appointed to institutions rather than elected have to find ways of

> The lay members in Hayes & Harlington were concerned that the members of the regular public panel were not representative of the local population. Consequently, they decided to engage in a broader outreach programme to local community groups. Through these meetings they undoubtedly encountered a wider range of voices, which did have an impact on their own views. But such one-off events could only have a marginal impact. It was the lay members' own voices and the voices of the public panel and the community health council which were heard by the board, because they were confident, sustained and aware of the corporate agenda. Without investment in building the confidence of distant voices, this tension is inescapable.

I can't represent everybody in the community, but I can tell them the experience I've got through being in the voluntary sector which actually provides care in the community, that actually is in touch with carers and people with local care needs. Maybe we could have done something around getting people's opinions about how they felt PCGs could have changed the way in which services are developed. But none of that has been done... none of it.

Lay member

speaking with authority and this typically requires speaking for others as well as yourself. Although most lay members distanced themselves from the 'representative' tag, they were all involved in speaking up for patient, carer and public interests. They were representing (i.e. advocating for) public interests, rather than being a representative of the local community. This sense of representation as advocacy comes closest to the role that lay members performed.

The lay members in our case studies brought varying degrees of knowledge and experience of the local community to their roles. There was a very clear relationship between this knowledge and their authority as lay members. Those who had plenty of local knowledge and experience working with local people were the most confident and most able to speak with authority. Those who had little knowledge and experience found it very hard to establish a role and voice among their professional peers. Those who actively engaged in public involvement work found that this was itself a means to gaining credibility as lay voices as well as personal confidence.

Whose agenda?

For primary care organisations, public involvement is about bringing two sets of interests together in some way: the interests of the public and the interests of the organisation and its professionals. Involvement work will only produce meaningful results if these two sets of interests can serve each other.

If either side of this equation is ignored, you get something other than public involvement. If patient, carer and public interests are ignored, you end up with the worst kind of public relations – a process of organisational legitimation that exploits rather than values public input. If corporate interests are ignored you either end up with an involvement process which goes nowhere because no-one in the organisation is interested or community development, i.e. a process of change which is defined and led by the community.

Public involvement is not community development, though community development may play a crucial role in enabling public involvement. If a primary care

One of the reasons I had applied for the job was that I had worked with families and young people all from this area so I felt that I really knew what was happening in a lot of people's homes and families and what their cares and worries were. A lot of the things are not health but they are all inter-related like poor housing, family problems, and things like that that are all linked in the end. I would like to feel that I can become more conversant with what the people in the area want so that I am then able to have a stronger voice on the board – a more convinced voice possibly rather than just my own personal thoughts and feelings.

Lay member

The community is quite critical of our lack of input or our failure to make a space within which they could input. Although there is an acknowledgement that we mustn't expect people to come to us and that we need to go to them, our workloads are such and the challenges around working with such a diverse – culturally and linguistically diverse – community are absolutely enormous.

Officer

The Central Croydon community network meetings were an explicit attempt to bridge corporate and public interests. The formal agenda was largely set by the organisation and included items of corporate business. But the diversity of people who came ensured that many other concerns were raised. The challenge for the lay member was to get useful feedback on the corporate issues while also respecting and addressing, as far as possible, the issues which were raised by participants. The danger was always that in trying to do both, neither would get enough time for proper consideration. This is a struggle for all such enterprises.

Service users and community care: new roles, new knowledges, new forms of involvement?

Beresford P. *Managing Community Care* 2000; vol. 8 no. 6: 20–23.

Beresford argues that it is precisely because users have different agendas and interests from providers that their voices are so powerful. He identifies five key ways in which the perspectives of community care users are likely to be different from 'traditional stakeholders':

- Different knowledges, based both on experience of the problem which defines their community care need and on experience of being a user.
- Different interests and objectives, including challenging oppression and improving quality of life.
- Different philosophies, values and ideas, such as a rights-based rather than needs-based approach to public policy and personal assistance.
- Different ways of doing things, particularly through collective rather than individual action.
- Different forms of communication, including sign and picture-based languages.

All these differences present challenges for providers, but they are constructive challenges. There are, however, two further differences which are always obstacles: differences in power and legitimacy:

> 'Service users and their organisations have significantly less power and the funding that goes with it than service providers and policy-makers… Unequal weight is generally attached to the different knowledges and perspectives of service providers and users. This is a general issue, but it applies particularly to groups like mental health service users/survivors and people with learning difficulties, the validity of whose perceptions, judgements and intellects are routinely called into question.'

User groups are often perceived by providers to be relatively easy to reach in public involvement work. Crucially, the challenge for providers is not only in reaching the voices of users, but in respecting and valuing all the differences which inform user perspectives. The greatest challenges may come from the strongest collective voices.

In our case studies, there were few examples of direct dialogue between providers and users which fully exploited the differences in their perspectives. This was principally because of the lack of direct engagement with strong collective voices. Often, a piece of public involvement work would be followed by professional consideration of the 'results', thereby losing the power of the direct encounter. When direct encounter did occur, it was usually with a range of fragmented voices, rather than with a clear shared perspective.

organisation is to value, use and respond to patient, carer and public voices, it has to attend to its own agenda as well as to the agenda of those it is communicating with. This creates a tension that is played out in a wide variety of ways in all public involvement work.

Successful public involvement relies on bridging institutional and public interests. This also means bringing world views together in a meaningful way. This is not an easy process as a willingness to listen, think differently and compromise is needed on both sides. Too much emphasis on the organisation's agenda and lay people may feel ignored, exploited or simply confused. Too much emphasis on a community agenda and an organisation may find itself with a long list of actions that it has no power to deliver on. The more an organisation seeks to engage with its user and public partners on their terms, the more it is likely to need the support of a partnership approach to public involvement in order to do something meaningful with what it hears.

In our case studies, the primary care organisations struggled to get this balance right. There is no single answer. For example, some of the organisations invested in 'deliberative' methods in which lay people were given time and resources to develop their understanding of institutional interests and decision-making, thereby bringing them closer to an understanding of the organisation's agenda. Alternatively, some pursued outreach methods or events with open agendas in which members and officers tried to engage with local people on their own terms. Both approaches have their problems: the former can fail to pick up on the priorities of local people; the latter relies on a clear (but often absent) process of making the connections to organisational change after the event.

Although it is difficult to design processes that 'meet in the middle' effectively, such meetings take place all the time. At a personal level, members, officers, professionals, patients, carers and local people are always meeting, talking, arguing and, hopefully, changing the way they view the world. Openness to difference, surprise and new ideas is not so unusual.

Say you are asking something like 'what should the prescribers' budget be for the PCG in the three year plan?' Well, if you're going to a group of refugees who maybe haven't got anywhere to live permanently, let alone any money to spend on healthy food, and enormous mental health problems, then that's not really a priority for them, what the three year plan looks like. I don't mean that their issues shouldn't inform what's in the three-year plan but you have to start somewhere else.

Officer

People have to get their head round the way in which people talk about the health authority in foreign language. I went to a meeting on Wednesday and there's somebody there talking about critical mass. I understand the concept of critical mass but, do me a favour, they were talking about one person as the critical mass. I mean critical mass sounds like an illness.

Lay member

At a meeting of the Harrow East & Kingsbury board, a visiting consultant found himself having something of an argument with the GPs who were frustrated with their difficulties and delays in getting referrals and the problems with communication. However, the consultant knew how to handle fellow professionals: he simply deflected their complaints by describing the hospital's own problems in communicating with local GP practices. Then two women in the public seats were invited to speak. They tore into the consultant, telling him that the delays and mistakes with referrals were completely unacceptable. The consultant was literally at a loss for words. When he could no longer play the professional game, he had no defence to fall back upon. He had to take the criticism seriously.

Chapter nine

Making a difference

KEY POINTS

The structure of primary care organisations does not
enable them to learn 'as a matter of course' from patient
and public voices.

Emphasis on external mechanisms of involvement easily
leads to a neglect of the internal mechanisms of change.

The formal decision-making process works through
argument and persuasion. Public voices need advocates at
the heart of these debates.

Beyond the formal decision-making process, influence is
maximised through personal contact between officers, or
members and local people.

Public involvement work is likely to have its greatest
impact if it connects to existing processes of change
within primary care organisations.

The single biggest criticism made of public
involvement work by professionals and lay people
alike is that it fails to bring about change. It simply
doesn't make any difference.

There are plenty of easy targets for this criticism:
consultations that are carried out after the key
decisions have been made; high-profile initiatives
designed solely to demonstrate corporate credentials;
patient forums which are used to rubber stamp policy
decisions. But this criticism can also be levelled at
much of the public involvement work that is driven
by genuine interest in patient and public views.

The problem is not simply that people in institutions
are disinterested in change (although this is a very
real problem in itself) but that achieving change
through public involvement is far from easy and
certainly not straightforward. This chapter explores
these problems, describing:

- an institutional view of how NHS organisations
  learn and change
- the potential for improving the system to make it
  more responsive to public views

- alternative understandings of how change is achieved
- the challenge of connecting public involvement to the heart of organisational change
- the immediate results for patients, carers and public along the way.

An institutional view of the NHS

People who work within the NHS tend to assume that the structure within which they work operates as it should. Of course, there are lots of political shenanigans, but there is still a certain way of doing things that brings about change. Primary care organisations have boards for which papers get written and where key decisions get made. The members are accountable for the decisions, but the officers do most of the leg work in shaping the final form of policy. For all the informal influences upon officers and members alike, the basic process holds up.

Many of the people in our case studies implicitly or explicitly accepted this view. For them, the task was to ensure that public involvement work had an impact within this system. However, there were very different perceptions of the nature of this task. Some felt that the system had to be shaken up a bit if it was going to respond to public involvement work (see next section); others were reasonably comfortable with things as they were.

Those who accepted things as they were tended to focus their energies on the mechanisms of involvement rather than the mechanisms of change – they assumed the latter were in reasonable working order. This is characteristic of much public involvement work: lots of attention paid to the up-front process of involvement; much less attention paid to how the back-end process of change actually delivers. This assumes that there is an almost automatic process of learning which organisations are designed to sustain: outcomes from involvement initiatives get written up; the report goes to the board; members read the report; the report is debated; considered decisions emerge.

Unfortunately, this rarely happens. In practice, board members are overwhelmed with papers which they always receive late; they barely have time to read the

In trying to formulate our overall strategy, part of it would be saying 'well, if we find out such and such information what do we do with it?' Then I guess it has to come to the board, which would hopefully, where possible, make changes in service provision. However, if it's down to individual practices there's a limit to what you can do to individual practices. You can encourage them, but the amount to which the board can control what practice X does is limited.

Lay member

The Service and Financial Framework as a document was just totally naff anyway. You've got 60 priorities. The PCG really wanted to keep it to ten. That's what they set themselves, that's what we said to the public. It's like we don't want the shopping list, we want to say this is what our PCG will do – seven to ten things. And, of course, by the time it all got amalgamated with what the health authority wanted we were up to 60 something, because you've got your national priorities, your local priorities, your HImP priorities… all of these different conflicting priorities. But we took it to the forum and there has been dialogue. Like the diabetes people who were concerned about eye screening, that has got moved up. There have been minor influences in that way.

Officer

Developing learning organisations in the new NHS

Davies H and Nutley S. *BMJ 2000*; vol. 320: 998–1001.

Why is it so difficult for NHS organisations to learn from user and public voices? Why is it so difficult for NHS organisations to learn? Davies and Nutley provide a concise introduction to the key features of the 'learning organisation' in the context of contemporary NHS policy.

Organisational learning can be described at three levels:

- 'single loop learning', i.e. maintaining a steady course by identifying and addressing errors
- 'double loop learning', which opens the organisation to changes of course – redefining goals, norms, policies, procedures or structures
- 'learning about learning', building on the experience of learning to develop and test new learning strategies.

The NHS tends to get stuck at the first level, so established are its ways of doing things. The second level is far more challenging and typically requires 'unlearning' of existing practice as well as the creation of new approaches. Only if this more radical approach to learning is accepted will 'learning about learning' become meaningful and productive.

In our case studies, advocates of public views constantly came up against organisations unable to face the challenge of 'double-loop learning'. Yet it is here that the potential of public involvement lies: in rethinking systems and priorities rather than simply getting existing systems to run properly on their rails. Each of the primary care organisations was necessarily coping with a huge amount of change, but most professionals wanted to minimise the disruption this caused, rather than grasping yet more opportunities for changing their practice and organisation.

Davies and Nutley identify the following as integral to a learning organisation: celebration of success; absence of complacency; tolerance of mistakes; belief in human potential; recognition of tacit knowledge; openness; trust; outward looking. They note that:

> 'some of these values – for example, the celebration of success – are already central to the healthcare professions and the NHS, while others such as openness and trust may need more work'.

Public involvement is itself an integral part of the process of building openness and trust. This was acknowledged corporately in two of our case studies. In both, there was some recognition that although current public involvement work struggled to have an impact, it contributed to the longer-term development of an organisation which would be able to value and learn from user and public voices.

critical papers in any depth; the papers on public involvement are way down the agenda and only get a cursory glance; the findings from public involvement initiatives get their own slot, unconnected to the rest of the organisation's business; time and energy is running out when the slot is reached; there is little incentive for members to take the views seriously, given everything else they have to think about; a few congratulatory words are said and the chair moves the meeting on.

Both of these descriptions of board process are caricatures. The latter is a collation of typical problems, not a typical event. But it illustrates the basic problem. Formal mechanisms may be necessary for making formal decisions, but they are not designed as opportunities for people to listen, reflect and learn. Because user and public views do not sit easily within technical business agendas, they are particularly difficult to assimilate, value and use effectively within these contexts.

Improving the system

If NHS organisations do not respond well to patient, carer and public views, how can they be improved?

One important improvement was introduced with primary care groups: the lay member. Although NHS trusts have always had non-executive directors with a brief to represent community interests, lay members were much more focussed on this responsibility, not least because they usually had a leadership role in public involvement (see page 38). Many lay members not only kept the user/public interest alive in board and subgroup discussions, they also advocated broader public involvement initiatives by ensuring that reports, minutes and notes from such initiatives were received, read and duly considered. As such, they became a central mechanism for organisational learning from public involvement.

This was, however, an extremely difficult task. Given the pressure on PCG agendas, it was not easy for lay members to get their peers to attend to the importance of what lay people elsewhere were saying. In two of our case studies, the lay members were responsible for 'feeding back' to the board the views of standing user/public forums. This was an almost

> In Hayes & Harlington, the lay members were active at every level of the corporate process. As well as attending board meetings, they also sat on board subgroups and inevitably got caught up in the day-to-day life of the organisation. In their experience, the influence they exerted on the organisation was inversely proportional to the formality of their engagement with it. Once papers had got to the board, all the hard work had been done, so there was much less scope for influence. There was much more scope for real impact through working on the subgroups in the development of papers and communicating on a regular basis with the officers.

> *So I think our approach is to ask: 'Right, well, where do your decisions get made?' Well, they get made when you're developing the document involved. Well, how can we involve people at that stage? We tried to have, in theory, meetings about how to write that document, recognising that the actual decision period is during its writing as well as when it gets to the board.*
>
> **Chair**

impossible task, given the diversity of views that they had to summarise and communicate. Inevitably, the passion of the original speakers got lost in the process.

Lay members helped, but the system was still dominated by professional interests and priorities, not very 'fit' for dealing effectively with user and public views. The management of board meetings illustrated the problem. In most of our case studies, the primary care organisation made some effort to make their board meetings more open and accessible to members of the public. Yet despite these efforts, hardly any members of the public ever turned up (in all cases). Why should they? They were meetings held in public, not public meetings. The papers were technical, the business was oriented to provider interests not public interests and there was no place in the debate for individual experience. It would take considerable effort and imagination, let alone commitment, to run a primary care organisation's board meetings in a way that was really open to public views.

The formal process of decision-making basically works through argument, debate and persuasion. The more people there are within this debate to advocate for public voices, the more likely they are to bring about change. Other than lay members, the people who were able to do this in our case studies were community health council officers, some of whom had a long track record of contributing to board debates, and voluntary sector officers, usually through joint planning mechanisms. However, there were also insiders who were committed to listening to, and advocating for, public voices. On every board there were members who supported the lay member in pressing for greater attention to the lessons of public involvement. These included people from all professions, though nurses, social services and health authority non-executive members were the most prominent.

Alternative approaches to enabling change

Cranking up the formal system is not the only way to enable institutions to respond to public involvement. An alternative is to treat the institution as a messy,

In North Lewisham, the lay member introduced 'impact statements' to board papers. These required the officers and members writing the papers to describe what they though the potential impact of their proposals would be on the patients, carers and the public. The statements also required authors to describe any involvement work which had been undertaken in the development of the paper. In principle, this was a helpful way both of focussing minds on user/public interests and making the links between public involvement work and organisational change. However, thinking through these questions was not easy and there was no support available to do this. The statements risked becoming another bureaucratic hoop to get through.

How service users become empowered in human service organizations: the empowerment model.

Holosko M, Leslie D, Rosemary Cassano D. *International Journal of Health Care Quality Assurance* 2001; vol. 14 no. 3: 126–132.

By describing the involvement of users with health services in terms of empowerment, Holosko and his colleagues draw attention to the price of failure: disempowerment. If service providers do not value and use the views which they have solicited, their users are likely to feel even more pessimistic about their power to change institutional thinking.

> '*Turning the process of empowerment to one of disempowerment can occur at any level of the administrative process where service user input and its impact disappears into a "black hole".*'

This was borne out in our case studies, for example: in the chair of a patient participation group whose survey work was ignored by the GP; the lay member whose professional peers blanked her out on the board; the members of the public forum who had no idea of what, if anything, the PCG did with their recommendations. All these people experienced disempowerment, though they all persevered.

The authors describe a detailed framework for incorporating user input 'at all levels of the administrative continuum', emphasising the need for feedback and transparency. However, the model assumes that the key points of decision-making can all be identified in the quest for transparency:

> '*The closer the fit between service user expectations and decisions made, the higher the sense of empowerment. Similarly, the greater the discrepancy between service user expectations and decisions, the more important the need for shared information and explanation becomes.*'

In our case studies, failure to feedback about the user views was common. However, user views did not just impact on the formal points of decision-making, but on thinking, attitudes, practice and day-to-day decision-making throughout the primary care organisations. Although these impacts may never be amenable to transparent feedback, they are crucial to the overall outcomes of public involvement work.

political process in which influence is brought to bear all the time; where learning and change are achieved in many informal and often unpredictable ways.

This understanding does not ignore the formal structures of decision-making, but treats them as part of a much bigger process in which there are always opportunities emerging. The emphasis is on the ongoing dialogue between all stakeholders in a health economy that constantly informs individual learning, attitudes and practice. The task for those engaged in public involvement is to ensure that patient, carer and public views are always part of this dialogue, integral to the conversations, meetings, events and encounters which make up the fabric of an organisation's life.

This is a cultural understanding of change rather than a systems understanding. The aim is to get user and public views into the lifeblood of an organisation, rather than to identify the precise points in the process where their impact can be secured.

In our case studies, a variety of interpretations of this approach were expressed or pursued, in more or less explicit ways. The key feature in all of them was personal contact. Directly engaging members and officers in dialogue with lay voices, at any opportunity, was the key to ensuring that these voices were taken seriously. For example, in both of the case studies in which standing forums for public involvement were established, the system was supposed to work by lay members reporting views from the public forums to their boards. In practice, real influence was only achieved when other members and officers attended these forums themselves and engaged directly in debate with users and members of the public. These events were at a distance from the formal locus of decision-making, so it was not obvious exactly what impact these conversations would have on board decisions, but the potential for influence on the decision-makers was far greater.

The difficulty with this approach is its lack of transparency. It relies on quiet, often hidden, influence taking place all the time, rather than explicit processes where influence can be identified

In Harrow East & Kingsbury, diabetic support groups were run principally to inform and educate the patients who came along. However, the diabetic specialist nurse who ran them also played a critical role in picking up on personal concerns within the group discussions and, if appropriate, taking them to the relevant professionals at practice level. By maintaining good relationships with the practice nurses and, to a lesser extent, the GPs across the PCG, she was able to resolve individual problems and improve practice. She completely ignored the formal processes of decision-making and learning in the PCG but sustained a shared process of learning through her informal network of professional contacts.

The Chief Exec very often comes to the meetings and that's a definite factor. If members of the public can actually see that the Chief Exec is there they'll come, which is something we hope to keep going.

Voluntary sector officer

and measured. It therefore relies on political astuteness, on the ability of the people involved to identify and exploit opportunities wherever they can rather than expecting the system to work for them. However, this is not a mysterious process – it is principally about generating as many opportunities as possible for members and officers of primary care organisations to engage with patient, carer and public views; finding ways of bringing influence to bear on all existing ways of working.

One of the strengths of this perspective is the value it places on long-term cultural change. Changing professional attitudes and practice, developing new partnerships and new ways of working and communicating, creating open organisations – these outcomes rely on the slow feed of alternative views, not the occasional input to strategic decision-making.

Connecting to the change agenda

Whether you try to bring about influence through formal or informal mechanisms, through papers to the board or regular phone calls to the chief officer, your impact will still depend on whether you are pressing the right institutional buttons – whether you are connecting to the internal agenda for change.

Primary care organisations have, along with everyone else in the NHS, faced incredibly demanding change agendas. They have had to develop new approaches to service development and delivery; new forms of quality management; new relationships across old health economy boundaries; new approaches to commissioning and the prioritisation and use of resources; and new ways of thinking about and promoting local health. They have also had to deal with their own transformation from small health authority subgroups to independent NHS trusts.

This busy agenda is usually perceived as an obstacle to public involvement work. Yet wherever there is change, there are opportunities for influence. Unfortunately, public involvement work is more likely to be treated as yet another item on the change agenda than a key instrument in shaping the outcomes of the agenda as a whole. In our case studies, clear connections between organisational interests and the public involvement agenda were

In North Lewisham, a small community development organisation had a track record in working with local GP practices to identify and address community health needs. The director of this organisation took every opportunity she could to advocate for the communities she worked with. This meant spending time with the officers of all the local statutory authorities and identifying people who were responsive and willing to take community concerns seriously. This proved to be an easier task with local primary care groups than it had been with the more distant health authority.

Take repeat prescriptions. I'm on the prescribing subgroup and one of the things that we're really doing a lot of work on at the moment is repeat prescribing for patients. Now, we have not considered asking any users, constant users of medication, what they feel about the current process. What we've done is focused on practice managers and on GPs but the person at the other end who goes and collects it needs to be asked 'What is it like for you when you've been on long-term antidepressants?' I visit patients who go with their pre-printed prescription asking for one item but actually get prescribed the whole lot. They go to the pharmacy, the pharmacy is quite happy – he's making money out of it.

If there was a register of people, for instance, who had long-term drug therapy, then we could ring up and say 'Would you like to come to the surgery? We're actually having a meeting about repeat prescriptions and we'd really value what you've got to say about it.' But the GPs tend to see it as a purely organisational issue, but it isn't. It really, really isn't.

Nurse member

mainly limited to major, discrete projects. Little effort was made to systematically think through the potential for public involvement across the entire organisational change agenda. It is relatively easy to make these connections when a new project is launched with clear developmental goals and, typically, a strong service focus. It can be much harder to treat the on-going business of the organisation as raw material for public involvement.

There are clearly some parts of the primary care agenda that are more amenable to user and public input than others. Clinical governance, prescribing, commissioning and health improvement present more opportunities than performance management, financial monitoring and governance – though, ironically, it is the latter issues which are the traditional concern of non-executive directors. Yet, with a little imagination, there is potential almost anywhere.

Integrating public involvement into existing change agendas does not mean abandoning it as a separate agenda item. Unless there is very strong corporate leadership on the issue, this is more likely to lead to increased exclusion of public involvement from organisational interests. Yet, if the connections are not made with the rest of the agenda, its marginal status will remain and its impact will be limited.

In our case studies these connections were made in a variety of ways. Lay members were important, particularly when they sat on board subgroups for issues other than public involvement. Within these groups they could engage directly with the detailed business of the organisation, bring in user and public perspectives, and identify the value of further public involvement in addressing the specific agenda for change. Chief officers were also important. They had a clear overview of all the interests of the organisation and so were in a good position to identify where public involvement work could help progress these interests.

But most of the public involvement work was developed with relatively weak initial links to organisational interests. For example, several of the primary care organisations used the local Health Improvement Programme priorities to define

With mental health there is a working group within the PCG at the moment and there's a local African/Caribbean project that has done some work with people who have been diagnosed with mental health problems, using a community development approach focussing on what their needs are. And they've written up a report and they've got some very clear recommendations so it's a question of making sure that the report goes into the subgroup so that they start to look at how they might implement some of those recommendations, or how they might take it forward.

Officer

In Dagenham, the research project into the voices of vulnerable people began as an idea in the subgroup; although the board was informed about it, they had no particular reason to buy into it. As a piece of work exploring patient and community perspectives on health and social care needs, the danger was that it would fail to connect with the institutional concerns of the PCG. Nonetheless, when it was published, the officer responsible for taking it forward felt that it was extremely well placed to be taken seriously by the board. In particular, the new chief executive had a background in social services and the report was all about the need for integrated care; the new NSFs on older people and mental health had to be implemented and the report described the reality of local needs in these client groups; the NHS Plan made clear that the new PCT had to listen more carefully to patient views and this intervention demonstrated that the organisation had the ability to do this. However, it was up to this officer to make sure that these connections were made and sustained.

community consultation events. These events generated a wealth of ideas and views from local people, but it proved difficult to get the organisations to value these – the HImP was not as central to the pressing interests of the organisation as they had hoped.

It is, of course, important not to impose an organisational agenda on patients, carers and local people, but to find ways of connecting organisational interests with community interests – meeting half way. Public involvement should not be just a tool for solving organisational problems, but a process for articulating shared problems and shared solutions.

Outcomes along the way

This chapter has focussed on ways in which primary care organisations can achieve change through public involvement. Most public involvement work is geared to bringing about change in professional practice, service delivery or strategic decision-making. However, outcomes for patients, carers and local people do not all depend on organisational change happening first. There are plenty of immediate outcomes along the way.

Information and education work is, of course, designed to have a direct impact on the people who get involved. In almost every form of public involvement work, the people who get involved learn something as a direct result of participating, whether or not this is an intended outcome.

Public involvement work can deliver many other immediate outcomes, for patients, carers, local people, communities and voluntary sector organisations. Beyond improvements in knowledge, people may achieve greater confidence in dealing with professionals; greater confidence in managing their own health and illness; greater shared capacity to tackle community health issues; and greater understanding of how to make the system work for individual and community interests. There are also immediate outcomes for the professionals who get involved in doing the work – which may be more powerful than the impact of the final reports or other outputs.

In North Lewisham, the facilitator of a consultation day for older people presented the report from the day to the community participation subgroup, making a commitment to try and get the recommendations integrated into institutional strategic plans. However, the chair of the PCG was at the meeting and immediately identified an issue which was relevant to the current business of the prescribing group, which she also sat on. A direct connection had been made to the immediate interests of the organisation, thanks to the range of issues which the chair had to keep in her head all the time.

In Harrow East & Kingsbury, the public involvement subgroup did not spend much time thinking about how their work would bring about change. However, when the results of their survey of the local citizens' panel were presented to the board, they proved to be extremely timely, coinciding with board discussion of exactly the issues which the survey addressed. This was, to a degree, good fortune, but it also reflected the consistency with which the officers concerned had kept the issues which they knew were important to the PCG – access in particular – to the fore in the design of the survey (which took the better part of a year). They were not tempted to make the survey about 'everything they wanted to know', but kept a clear focus on their own organisational priorities.

Chapter ten

A range of approaches

There are lots of ways of going about public involvement work, and lots of methods to choose from. This chapter explores these choices, focussing on the types of approach rather than the detail of the methods.

Each of the approaches described here is not a complete account of what any primary care organisation might do. In our case studies, every primary care organisation drew on a combination of these approaches, depending on local circumstances, values and priorities.

This chapter is not comprehensive, but gives a flavour of the breadth of ideas and opportunities available to primary care organisations, covering:

- lay representation
- opening up the corporate process
- building relationships with the voluntary/ community sector
- standing mechanisms
- outreach
- one-off methods and interventions
- patient participation at practice level.

Lay representation

Lay members played a crucial role on primary care groups as institutional representatives of patient, carer and public interests. Lay members forced their professional peers to address the role of non-professional views in their work and decision-making. This encouraged a slow but sure shift in organisational culture which made more space for all forms of user and public voices.

Institutional lay voices can be powerful at any level of health service practice. People who understand the inside but bring the values and insights of the outsider provide a critical check on professional forgetfulness about who and what their services are for. But such roles require an 'expertise' all of their own. Lay voices should not be naïve voices, but

As a voluntary organisation, we develop things in the community via what people in the community are saying they need the most. That is done in a variety of ways: inviting people to speak to us as individuals, going out there and talking to them in their own homes, doing yearly surveys on how they find our services and what they want us to develop. There are lots of ways to do that; public involvement is a vast thing, it is not just saying 'well, we will put this particular thing and that's it, that's our public involvement'. Actually, it affects everything you do.

Voluntary sector officer

The whole issue of walk-in centres came up and it became very apparent that the majority of the board were unhappy about them. Probably got good reasons but I said 'well, hang on a minute, from my point of view, if I can just go down the road to get my ears syringed or have an injection or something in my lunch hour that's great, I don't have to take time off work, I don't have to rush, as far as I am concerned that is excellent'. So it's bringing a completely different point of view.

Lay member

voices of people who recognise the differences between professional interests and patient/public interests, people who can advocate for the experience of the user with an understanding of the priorities of the provider. The investment required to enable lay members to fulfil such a role, including training in the business of health care and in the challenges of public involvement, is easily underestimated.

In our case studies, the principal challenge for lay members was to gain respect and authority as full members of their boards. Some of the PCG boards welcomed the lay member from the outset, but acceptance did not ensure that their voices carried weight in discussion and decision-making. In order to gain authority, lay members had to demonstrate that they could contribute to organisational business in meaningful ways. They had to find the right balance between the voice of the insider, accepting the constraints, priorities and language of the organisation, and the voice of the outsider, challenging colleagues to think about their work and assumptions in different ways.

Lay members were most successful when they learned to play the corporate game but still continued to question the priorities which dominated institutional thinking. Training helped (in two cases studies), but this skill was largely acquired through the experience of debate on boards and sub-groups, where an in-depth knowledge of professional values was rapidly gained.

The non-executive director role on primary care trust boards is formally different from the primary care group lay member role, being more focussed on concerns of governance and probity. However, the tension between insider and outsider voices remains. Non-executive directors must pursue the organisation's interests while also being prepared to challenge those interests and question organisational priorities. It is unlikely that non-executive directors will be as closely involved in public involvement as lay members have been, but they still need to keep in touch with local community concerns if they are to fulfil their role fully.

In City & Hackney, the lay member was accepted and respected by other members of the PCG board. With considerable experience of the local voluntary sector, she was able to bring a detailed knowledge of the wider agenda of health – regeneration, housing, neighbour-hood renewal – and pressed other members to try and make the connections with this agenda. She did not try to represent the community, but made representations to the board about community needs and opportunities. In doing so, she was challenging the other board members not to think of her as a community voice, but rather to think more strategically in their decision-making about community needs.

In Dagenham, the lay member brought a great deal to her role: detailed knowledge of the needs of local people; extensive influence and contacts within the voluntary sector; experience of listening to and advocating for patient interests; and knowledge and experience of how organisations and institutions work. Yet the PCG board failed to value these resources. Crucially, when she first joined the board, she was not introduced properly or given a chance to explain what she had to offer. Simple procedural failings contributed to an on-going institutional failing to value lay voices.

In Hayes and Harlington, there was a clear distinction of roles between the lay members on the locality executive boards, who did not sit on the primary care trust board, and the trust non-executive directors. The lay members were responsible for (and actively pursued) public involvement work in their localities, whereas the non-executive directors focussed on corporate governance and had no special responsibility for public involvement. Nonetheless, the non-executive directors were expected to attend to what the lay members were hearing in order to fulfil their own roles as 'critical friends' more effectively.

Toolkits and good practice guides

The following is a selection of practical guides to public involvement. These titles were all in print or available on the internet when this publication went to press.

Barker J, Bullen M, de Ville J. *Reference manual for public involvement.* London: Lambeth, Southwark and Lewisham Health Authority, 1999.

Carter T, Beresford P. *Age and change: models of involvement for older people.* York: Joseph Rowntree Foundation, 2000.

Chambers R. *Involving patients and the public: how to do it better.* Oxford: Radcliffe Medical Press, 1999.

Dunman M, Farrell C. *The POPPi Guide: practicalities of producing patient information.* London: King's Fund, 2000.

Fajerman L, Jarrett M, Sutton F. *Children as partners in planning – a training resource to support consultation with children.* London: Save the Children, 2000.

Listen up! Effective community consultation. London: Audit Commission, 1999.

McIver S. *Obtaining the views of black users of health services.* London: King's Fund, 1994.

McNeish D. *From rhetoric to reality – participatory approaches to health promotion with young people.* London: Health Education Authority, 1999.

Patient consultation and involvement. A toolbox for general practice. London: East London and The City Health Authority, 2000.

Primary health care teams. Involving patients: examples of good practice. London: NHS Executive, 1997.

Public engagement toolkit. Northern & Yorkshire NHS Executive
http://www.doh.gov.uk/nyro/pubtool.htm

Seargant J, Steele J. *Consulting the public: guidelines and good practice.* London: Policy Studies Institute, 1998.

Opening up the corporate process

Openness is not a traditional value of the health service. Yet this simple value describes a whole way of working which is properly part of public involvement work.

PCG board meetings were required to be held in public. This was one step towards openness which was challenging enough – many PCGs decided to intersperse their board meetings with 'seminars' and the like. There is clearly scope to go much further: opening a wider range of meetings to the public; developing accessible forms of communication about business and decision-making; bringing more outsiders into the internal process; ensuring that questions from local people and stakeholder organisations are answered with efficiency and honesty; setting targets and monitoring progress with transparency.

Such organisational developmental work aims to create an organisation which people can trust, engage with and relate to on a daily basis. This is more meaningful than public involvement work which reaches out to local people but then retires behind an organisational veneer when the critical decisions are made.

Much of the challenge of this approach lies in attention to detail. For example, in our case studies, board meetings were all fairly similar: they were all run as business meetings with very few members of the public present. Nonetheless, the approach of the chair always set the tone of the meeting and profoundly affected the ease with which members of the public could contribute. A warm welcome, board introductions, regular opportunities to contribute, and serious attention to questions when they were put – these all encouraged public engagement and promoted an image of the organisation as willing to listen.

The most important details always lie in how relationships are valued and managed. Trust and openness cannot be built without investment in relationships: with patients and public, with voluntary and community organisations, with professionals and staff. This may be one of the biggest challenges facing the health services, but this should not undermine the value of small, incremental steps.

In City & Hackney, considerable effort was put into building new relationships with local community organisations, professionals and other staff. This took time: most people were used to being ignored. Lots of little things helped: a chief officer who was willing to meet people on their own turf; an executive who answered questions rather than fending them off; a board which was willing to be open about how little it could actually change; and a commitment to communication across the whole health economy.

Building relationships with the voluntary/community sector

The voluntary and community sector is the most obvious and yet often most neglected resource for public involvement work. In every corner of the UK there are local organisations that bring people together to discuss and pursue their common interests. Some are large, well-organised and very well-off; others are small, precarious and entirely self-supporting. All of them are opportunities for institutional engagement with individual and community interests.

NHS professionals are often put off approaching community organisations because of fears that they will have 'special' interests or will not be representative. In practice, there are always problems deciding which organisations to invite to an event, consult with, or speak to. However, difficulty making such choices is never grounds for not making them at all.

Few community organisations have the capacity or willingness to engage with statutory bodies on a regular basis, so it is unlikely that a wide invitation will result in a primary care organisation being 'inundated'. It is important to select appropriate organisations to work with where possible, but this should be primarily driven by the aims of the consultation. If a primary care organisation is clear about its intentions, what it is seeking and what it hopes to do with what it gets, and it has good information about local organisations and their interests, the process of selection becomes transparent. Local umbrella groups can also play a crucial role in enabling and supporting this process.

The strength of community organisations is their collective nature. It takes considerable confidence as an individual to question the priorities of health professionals. Participation in a shared voice can therefore be empowering individually as well as collectively. It is this power which can be off-putting for professionals, particularly GPs for whom the one-to-one relationship is central to their practice.

In our case studies, voluntary and community sector organisations were valued in many ways: as collective voices of patient and public interests; as sources of intelligence about community needs; as partners in exploring and addressing those needs; as sources of expertise about public involvement; and as routes for communication with marginalised communities. However, attitudes varied – the voluntary sector was perceived both as a close partner in corporate planning and as an unruly mass of local groups.

Any engagement with the voluntary sector should be sensitive to the capacity and interests of local organisations. Some will be more enthusiastic and more able to work in partnership than others. In only one of our case studies was any serious capacity-building in the voluntary sector being undertaken. This took the form of community development work: networking local groups and supporting them to identify and address common interests. This is a slow process, but it helps to knit together an otherwise fragmented health economy.

Standing mechanisms

NHS institutions are remarkably fond of standing mechanisms of public involvement. If you work within an institution, it is easy to assume that institutional models are a good way of doing things. In practice, forums, panels, councils and networks all have a familiar range of institutional strengths and weaknesses.

The principal weakness of standing mechanisms is their marginalisation from the decision-making of the organisation. Although attention tends to focus on the constitution, recruitment and operation of standing mechanisms, their real problems lie in the dotted lines which connect them to the power centres of the organisation where the decisions get made. The dotted line is often a single individual, responsible for ensuring that the thoughts of one forum get taken seriously in the decision-making of another. Given the dominance of professional interests at the heart of decision-making, such mechanisms are unlikely to be very powerful. This was the core problem of the two standing mechanisms in our case studies. In both cases, the forums were most effective when the decision-makers came to the forum and engaged directly with public voices. Only then did they really have to engage with the alternative values and perspectives of patients and local people.

The public panel run for Hayes & Harlington by the community health council brought together individual patients with representatives from patient participation groups and tenants associations. The agenda was usually dominated by PCG business. However, papers were presented cold without any strong steer from the PCG about what comments would actually be useful to them. Without clear questions, it was difficult for the group to focus on producing clear answers. Discussions about the papers were complex and wide-ranging, but they tended not to produce strong messages which might actually have the power to influence the PCG. The lay members were put in a difficult position in having to feed back these discussions to the board. Nonetheless, the panel did provide an opportunity for the members to learn about the PCG and, increasingly, engage with it on its own terms. It enabled people who had strong views about patient experience to make sense of (and interact with) the service-side issues which shaped that experience.

Once a forum becomes part of the routine of organisational life, it loses some of its power to challenge and can take on a life of its own. At worst, it becomes a tool for the organisation to legitimate its own decision-making.

The principle strength of standing mechanisms lies in the opportunity they give people to develop informed and meaningful relationships with health service professionals. They give people a chance to gain confidence, grapple with institutional agendas and get to know the system and the key professionals within it. This enables organisations to engage in a relatively sophisticated level of regular debate with patients, carers and local people. They are much more likely to enable 'deliberative' involvement than one-off methods.

The challenge in the development of standing mechanisms is to ensure that when people gain a stronger voice and clearer understanding of organisational priorities, the organisation responds by valuing this extra critical edge and actively finding ways of maximising its influence. The temptation is always to become more defensive and try to manipulate, rather than respect, the power of such voices.

Outreach

One of the defining features of any public involvement work is the turf it is conducted on. Most initiatives either happen within primary care territory or on neutral ground. Either way, the experience for people participating is, physically, of having to get to a meeting or event. This means that participants expect such events to be defined by an agenda other than their own. And, in practice, this is almost always what happens.

The alternative is for the organisation to go to the people. Meeting people on their own turf can be challenging precisely because it means being open to the agenda and interests of the people you are engaging with. The protective boundary of the organisational agenda is lost.

However, the choice of whose agenda to work with always remains. Institutional agendas tend to be

What we've got to work at first of all is developing a knowledge base because when you're living and breathing it you are so far ahead of everybody else. So although there are always going to be new people, the participants actually become the givers of that information, they actually become able to talk about this sort of stuff to other people or to their members. Again, it doesn't happen overnight but that is the process you need to go through, especially with something like PCGs because most people still won't have heard of them.

Lay member

I wanted the panel to be a very informal place where people could really feel free about talking about their experiences and those of other people they knew, but at the same time we could train up to an extent so that they could receive the information and actually comment on it in a slightly knowledgeable way.

Community health council officer

The PCT consultation undertaken by City & Hackney was an attempt to engage with people about their priorities rather than simply imposing an institutional agenda. Crucially, this involved going to meet community groups and being literally part of their agenda, rather than expecting them to come to the institution. However, the discussions still began with a presentation for the PCG about what the forthcoming changes involved, thereby narrowing the terms of debate to the organisation's immediate interests. Consequently, the feedback they got principally concerned the perceived quality of local health services rather than the health needs of the communities they spoke to.

dominant, wherever people meet. But professionals stand more chance of suppressing these in favour of alternative agendas the further away they get from the places where their power is accepted. Wherever dialogue takes place, active effort is needed to bridge organisational and community interests (see page 62).

In only two of our case studies were attempts made to engage with people in their own time and on their own turf. In both cases, the people involved from the PCG found the experience rewarding and challenging. However, in both cases it was very difficult to find a way of communicating what was learnt to the PCG in such a way that it would be meaningful for the business of the organisation.

One-off methods and interventions

Focus groups, surveys, citizens' juries, consensus conferences, public meetings, research projects – these are the common currency of public involvement work. But they are not the heart and soul of public involvement work. Each of these methods has its strengths and weaknesses, but they should always be part of a bigger endeavour.

One-off methods are often (but not always) tied to specific organisational interests or agendas. This can be a great strength if it means that there is a clear policy target where the work can impact. Such targeted input is in contrast to the general remit of standing mechanisms which can struggle to make clear or powerful connections to organisational interests.

The danger of one-off projects is the brevity of their opportunity for impact. If they do not have an immediate influence, they rapidly lose their chance of achieving anything as the policy environment changes. Their impact can only be secured if there are people who continue to actively lobby for the results to be taken seriously by the organisation. This role needs to be considered at the beginning of the project, not on its completion.

In our case studies, four of the primary care organisations invested in specific time-limited pieces of public involvement work. The projects were

I don't think that the public consultation was up to much. The public meeting that I went to had maybe 30 people in the audience. There was the top bracket at the top table with an overhead projector and a room with appalling acoustics, and probably of the 30 people in the audience 20–25 of us were staff and probably about five real people. So it is very clear to me that in this area that doesn't work.

Officer

developed for a variety of reasons – some were clearly tied to organisational priorities, others emerged out of general discussion of public involvement work. In all cases, impact was most likely if outputs had direct relevance to existing agendas within the organisation, with identified individuals or groups able to take them forward in the institutional process (see page 62).

Patient participation at practice level

There is a long history of patient participation in general practice. Patient participation groups (PPGs) were the mainstay of patient involvement in primary care for decades prior to the creation of primary care groups. However, the advent of primary care organisations has shifted the focus elsewhere: the members and officers of these corporate bodies have usually found it easier to develop their own public involvement work rather than try to nurture patient participation among their constituent practices. Nonetheless, this remains an important part of the public involvement agenda for primary care, as it keeps frontline primary care professionals in the dialogue with patient and public voices. This is crucial to the long-term goal of shifting professional practice towards a model of partnership.

Patient participation does not begin with PPGs but with the individual relationships between professionals, patients and carers. Patient participation at practice level will only prosper if there is professional willingness to change these relationships, to reach beyond the security of professional power to a more meaningful engagement with the values, interests and needs of the individual user. Although this relationship has not been a subject of this book, it lies at the heart of professional commitment to public involvement. If professionals do not see the value of partnership at the individual level, they are unlikely to value public involvement at the corporate level – though experience of the latter may shift perceptions of the former.

In our case studies, practice-level patient participation only flourished where there was enthusiasm on both sides: among both providers and users. Attempts to promote patient participation were foiled both by the wariness of professionals and

Much of the inspiration for Dagenham's public involvement work came from the Gables patient participation group. A key reason why the PPG flourished was its focus on relationships: between professionals and patients, and between all those with a connection to the practice as members of a shared community. PPGs are often set up as mechanisms for the patients to inform the professionals about their practice and services, or for professionals to educate their patients; either way, there is an imbalance in the contribution of each role. By emphasising changes in relationships and the promotion of community, the Gables PPG ensured that everyone took a shared responsibility for making the PPG a success.

In Central Croydon, the link person scheme was designed to connect the interests of patients in local practices to the interests of the PCG. It was successful for the PCG as a means of communicating with local practice populations, but it proved difficult to enable the communication the other way. Very few practices had patient participation groups, leaving most link patients without a collective forum to articulate the interests of practice users. It was very difficult for them to lobby the PCG for change when their individual appeals were not supported by any broader collective voice.

In North Lewisham, a local community development organisation had a long track record of working in general practice and encouraging public involvement. Their strategy was always to deal rapidly with professional fears by showing them how public involvement could benefit them. Initial needs assessment work almost always demonstrated high levels of support among the patients – essential to winning the professionals over – as well as pointing to potential for change which the organisation's officers would help to enable. The PCG wanted quicker results, but found that not doing the persuasive groundwork risked losing the support of the professionals for the involvement process as a whole.

Patient participation groups in general practice in the NHS

Brown I. *Health Expectations* **1999; vol. 2: 169–178.**

Ian Brown describes the history of patient participation groups (PPGs) in the NHS and the findings of research into PPGs over the past thirty years. He identifies five key issues:

- the diversity of purposes pursued by PPGs
- the uneven distribution of PPGs, with fewer established in areas of greatest health need
- the unrepresentative membership of PPGs
- the difficulty of sustaining PPGs, given the high level of public disinterest
- the difficulty of assessing their costs and benefits.

Although we did not study the PPGs in our case studies in great detail, we can certainly concur with the first of these points. Like public involvement work in general, PPGs are a method which serves multiple aims. The particular direction any PPG takes will reflect the interests and power of the professionals and users involved locally.

The other points are likely to be perennial: PPGs can only thrive where there is local interest and, as Brown indicates:

> 'it seems likely that PPGs are a model that suit some people in the community and not others'.

It may be more fruitful to see PPGs as pockets of local community action rather than as policy solutions which require equity and representative membership in their delivery.

by the disinterest of patients. Enthusiastic patients and carers found that practice staff had neither the time or inclination to work with them; and enthusiastic professionals found themselves unable to recruit enough people to sustain a group.

The handful of PPGs across the case studies had very different priorities. The direction taken by any PPG inevitably depended on the interests and influence of both the lay and professional members. Some were geared to patient education; others to improving the quality of the service. The traditional focus on fund-raising was sustained in a minority. However, in only two instances was there any active effort by PPG members to engage with the broader interests of the primary care organisation.

Chapter eleven

Past and future

This study of six primary care organisations took place six years after a study of public involvement in six health commissions (see over). The consistency of the results from the two studies is striking. Every one of Lupton and Taylor's observations is supported by our work.

Primary care groups were much smaller organisations than health commissions. There was less capacity in their executives and they were more dependent on the unique role of the lay member. But structurally the contexts were very similar. Like health commissions, primary care groups were struggling with a new corporate role in a context of major upheaval; they were trying to make local sense of increased national policy emphasis on public involvement; they were struggling to shift the values of professional culture when the priorities of the short-term dominated; they were reaching out to public voices while trying to get to grips with their own capacity for change.

Six years on, are we back to square one? Is the NHS trapped in a routine of forgetfulness and re-invention in which professional interests always win out? Or is this just the latest turn in a path which does lead, albeit slowly, to ever-wider acceptance of the value of user and public voices?

It is perhaps inevitable that the ceaseless re-organisation of the NHS has damaged the development of public involvement work, which requires continuity and stability to prosper. You cannot build meaningful relationships if your identity is always changing. But, hopefully, the latest re-organisation has not been in vain. Primary care trusts, with unified budgets, responsibility for health improvement, close operational links with primary and community health services and duties of both partnership and public involvement, *ought* to be in a good position to build relationships with users, local people and local communities. If they retain the local focus that characterised primary care groups, and do not become another bunch of distant, corporate NHS institutions, they stand a chance of gaining respect as valued partners among the many other players in every local health economy.

Primary care groups were new corporate opportunities for public involvement in primary care. Primary care trusts present even greater opportunities: to build a new kind of NHS institution, based on openness and partnership, integral to the common efforts of communities to tackle illness and promote health.

This study has emphasised a cultural understanding of public involvement in which every relationship counts. We encourage primary care trusts:

- to value all their relationships, internal and external, with user and public voices: the formal and the informal; the strategic and the operational; the institutional and the casual; the systematic and the day-to-day
- to value the diversity of user and public voices, and the ambiguity of public involvement work
- to attend to how they learn and change from user and public voices, and to value all forms of learning, not just the formal mechanisms

- to bring user and public voices and their advocates into as many discussions and debates within the organisation as possible.

As lay members disappear, primary care trusts need to consider how to sustain public voices in all their business and decision-making. Public involvement should be just that: involvement, not just a process for generating information which then gets considered by professionals elsewhere. The NHS will only lose its fear of openness if it risks openness – and welcomes other voices in.

Coming in from the cold

Lupton C and Taylor P. *Health Service Journal*, 16th March 1995.

Lutpon and Taylor describe the results of a study of public involvement in the six health commissions of Wessex region. Interviews with chief executives and senior staff were undertaken in 1994, two years after the publication of *Local Voices*, which urged greater public participation in the commissioning process. The following are some of their observations:

- Senior managers all stressed corporate commitment to public involvement but accepted that it was frequently displaced by more urgent business.
- There was uncertainty in all commissions about the aim of public involvement and, in practice, it fulfilled diverse objectives.
- Work with service users on service-specific agendas was easier than broader engagement with the public, but staff struggled to render the information generated meaningful to the commissioning process.
- In the absence of clear organisational strategies, public involvement work was characterised by a 'pick and mix' approach.
- Significant organisational change made it difficult to sustain public involvement initiatives.
- The location of the public involvement brief within the organisation determined its focus. However, there was a growing recognition that public involvement had to move away from a 'project' mould to become integrated into all purchasing activity, to become 'everyone's business'.
- Staff with relevant past experience were more likely to express concerns and frustration with the work than those who had newly taken on the public involvement brief.
- The demands of national policy tended to skew public involvement work towards short-term, identifiable outcomes, undermining the development of more substantial ongoing forms of engagement.
- Lead staff often felt isolated and had to strive continuously to build understanding and support for public involvement within the organisation.

Overall, development of public involvement was enabled by the understanding and commitment of senior managers; the confidence and skills of lead staff; and positive organisational culture with effective internal mechanisms for using the messages from consumers and the public.

Chapter twelve

Appendix: methods

Selection of case studies

When the study began in February 2000, there were 66 primary care groups in London. Our approach to selection was to try and recruit as diverse and interesting a sample as possible. As this was a qualitative study, our concern was not that the cases should be representative, but that they should give us a breadth and depth of experience and ideas.

There were three grounds for exclusion prior to selection:

- if the PCG was participating in the national Tracker survey, in order to minimise research demands on busy people (10 exclusions)
- if no response had been received from either the chief executive or the lay member to our initial survey of public involvement in London's PCGs (see page 4) (one exclusion, also a Tracker site)
- if the survey response indicated that commitment to developing public involvement at board level was low and there was little evidence of completed or planned activity (10 exclusions).

Selection from the remaining 46 PCGs was designed to achieve the following similarities and differences:

- three with high deprivation indices (Department of Environment [DoE] index of local conditions between 20 and 40); three with low deprivation indices (DoE index between -20 and 0)
- three with minority ethnic populations greater than 25 per cent; three with minority ethnic populations less than 25 per cent
- three with populations greater than 100,000; three with populations less than 100,000
- three with intentions to move to PCT status by April 2001; three with longer-term expectations
- at least two with approaches to public involvement which included community development.

Almost all criteria were met, although only one of the two PCGs with an interest in community development proved to be engaging in anything substantial. Only two of the cases had populations of less than 100,000, but one of the other four had a population of 101,000.

Initial interviews

In each case study, we began research with a round of in-depth interviews with key individuals with an interest in public involvement. These varied between the cases but always included the lay member and a senior officer, often the chief officer. We also interviewed PCG chairs and other board members, community health council officers, voluntary sector officers and patient participation group members. The interviews were recorded and transcribed, with the permission of the interviewees.

Observation and participation

Following the initial exploratory work, we sought to tailor each case study to local interests. This involved discussions with local stakeholders about their priorities and the contribution which the study could make to their work.

Most of the ongoing research activity involved observation of meetings and initiatives. These included board meetings, public involvement subgroup meetings, user panel meetings and major public involvement events.

To varying degrees, this involvement went beyond observation to participation. This included contributions to discussion, assistance with research methods and limited support with facilitation of events. This level of participation enabled closer observation and deeper understanding of the complexity of local approaches to public involvement.

Although the initial interviews were crucial in describing the breadth of local interests and values, the (participant) observation was at the heart of the study. Given the opportunity, people are more than keen to talk about public involvement at length. But the challenge of public involvement is inevitably the translation of ideas and enthusiasm into practice.

Analysis and synthesis

The analysis drew on a diversity of data in each case study: the interview transcripts; observation notes from meetings and events; and local documents.

Drawing on the model of evaluation described by Ray Pawson and Nick Tilley (*Realistic Evaluation*, London: Sage, 1997) we were keen to explore the complexity of the local contexts which shaped the implementation and outcomes of public involvement work. However, because 'public involvement' is not a clear programme with clearly defined aims, but a broad value-based agenda with diverse outcomes, it proved difficult to define a rigorous approach to evaluation. Although lots of people had ideas about what they wanted to achieve, these were always changing and being renegotiated. We therefore focussed on the generic process of change, valuing any outcomes, whether intended or not.

Individual case study reports were produced for each primary care organisation. These were structured around a modified form of Pawson and Tilley's model (see over). The elements of this model are as follows:

- Context: history, demography, politics and people: the things which, even if they are open to change, are not matters of choice at the outset.
- Approach: the general terms of local engagement – why, how and for whom public involvement is pursued, but not the specification of methods.
- Mechanisms of involvement: the methods PCGs employ to involve patients and the public.
- Mechanisms of change: the ways in which PCGs bring about change in response to involvement initiatives.
- Outcomes: the impact of the mechanisms of involvement on PCGs, patients and local communities, encompassing a chain of impacts from the immediate impact of dialogue on participants, through PCG decision-making to improvements in the health and well-being of local people.

This model provided a means of identifying the particular forms of local activity within a common framework. Any explanation of public involvement requires an understanding of all these aspects of the model: of the particularity of the context and the approach(es) adopted; of the performance of the specific mechanisms used; and of the nature and importance of the outcomes achieved.

This publication is the synthesis of the research, drawing on the six case study analyses. Although the case studies were very diverse, we have sought to make connections across them in ways which we hope are illuminating for public involvement work in general. Although local contexts are always critical in defining what actually goes on, we believe that the issues raised in this publication are likely to be relevant for anyone pursuing public involvement in primary care organisations.

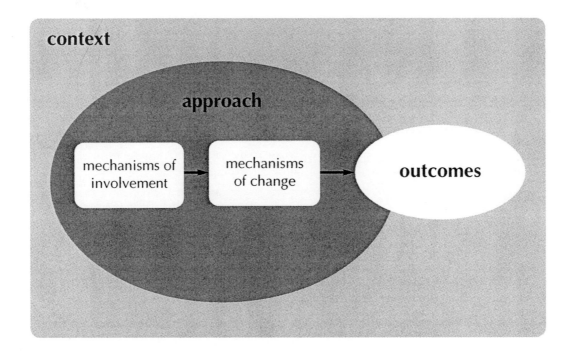